Praise for
Lessons of the Cards

"Hazel Curtis provides a unique approach to emphasizing the importance of keeping the "heart" in the healthcare profession. Her "all in the cards" metaphor will guide you through 10 secrets of igniting your passion while serving your patients."

G. Eric Allenbaugh, Ph.D., MPH
Wake-Up Calls and Deliberate Success

"To learn from Hazel is both educating and inspiring! She draws from her rich experience to identify key principles of caregiving. She understands the frustrations and demands of being a healthcare professional but provides hope in the form of *Lessons of the Cards*. With creative force, she explores today's healthcare challenges and provides meaningful ways to navigate them."

Kathy McMillan, RN, MA, Employee Spiritual Care

"*Lessons of the Cards*, by Hazel Curtis, will inspire many. A gifted speaker, a dedicated healthcare professional, and a seasoned leader, Curtis brings much wisdom and experience to this book. I hope it is read by many."

Gerald R. Winslow, PhD; Professor of Religion and Christian Bioethics
Loma Linda University

"In the decade that I have worked internationally with Hazel Curtis, I've seen the wisdom in her eyes, listened to the passion of her teaching and writing, and experienced her dedication to healthcare excellence. *Lessons of the Cards* is filled with useful information to bring respectful, dignified, compassionate care into a world of suffering."

Liana Yang, RN, PhD; Education Consultant
Hangzhou, China

"Hazel has done it! She has written a practical book for leaders navigating the transformations necessary in healthcare. And, she's used a deck of cards; how practical can you get? She provides valuable lessons learned through the various aspects of her healthcare career. The lessons are fun and resonate in a common language that remind us to laugh and persevere. After all, "Every Day, Life Deals You a New Hand!" Thank you, Hazel for sharing your life lessons, giving us some great tools, and providing heartfelt moments as well as laughter."

Dora Barilla, DrPH
A New Day: A True Story of Healing, Faith and Miracles

"Discovering the 10 secrets hidden in a deck of cards will ignite your resilience to persist in a healthcare world filled with patients, pressure, and promise. Your future can be bright!"

Caitlin Williams, Licensed Marital & Family Therapist
Kaiser Permanente

"This is a must read for healthcare professionals! Hazel Curtis takes us on a pragmatic and sometimes humorous journey through the ever-changing climate of our healthcare system. With her in-depth perception of the challenges, along with her genuine compassion, she draws our attention to why we chose our professions in the first place. Overall, the book inspires you to never lose sight of the art of healing as well as brings to light what a privilege it is to care for people in their most vulnerable times."

Elaine Hart, MD; Professor of Obstetrics and Gynecology
Loma Linda University School of Medicine

"Hazel's new book is chock full of useful information for nurses, physicians, and all healthcare providers. Her candid, no-holds-barred advice and real-life storytelling is a powerful combination bound to strike a chord with healthcare providers everywhere."

Claudia Cooley
The Seven Mind Shifts to Ignite your Success, and Revving Up for Success Series

LESSONS
OF THE CARDS

A GUIDE FOR HEALTH PROFESSIONALS

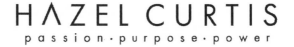

HAZEL CURTIS
passion · purpose · power

© 2019 by Hazel Curtis

Published by Hazel Curtis
Riverside, California
Printed in the United States of America

Cover illustration and design by Whitney Wolff
Interior design by Whitney Wolff

Library of Congress Cataloging-in-Publication Data
Curtis, Hazel 1950-
Lessons of the Cards: A Guide for Healthcare Professionals / Hazel Curtis.
ISBN 978-0-9996841-0-8
ISBN 978-0-9996841-1-5 *ebook*

1. Medicine 2. Personal Transformation 3. Life Coaching

Visit www.hazelcurtis.com

Requests for information should be addressed to: inspire@hazelcurtis.com

Dedication

This book is dedicated to the nurses who blazed the path to my success, most particularly:

Miss Emma Binder, RN 1901–1993   RN–1929; BSN–1947

Miss Alma Binder, RN   1911–2004   RN–1934; BSN–1946

Mrs. Darlena Stanford Voegele 1929–   RN, BSN–1952

Acknowledgment and Appreciation

I am deeply indebted to my Binder-Voegele-Curtis family, many who followed the call to serve in healthcare—physicians, dentists, therapists, nurses, paramedics, administrators-- you continually inspire and amaze me. We are so blessed to be family.

Finally, I wish to acknowledge all my colleagues— you know who you are! Whether a classmate, a coworker, or a participant in my audience—it is truly you who have made me a better practitioner, teacher, and coach. You have called my bluff, beat me hands down, trumped me, and partnered with me. Together we hold accountability, perseverance, and dedication to the healing arts as a sacred trust. Together we start conversations that change tomorrow. We've ranted, we've yelled, we've struggled, and we've cried. And, we are not nearly done yet!

Deep appreciation is extended to: The book-writing masterminds who brought out the best in me—especially Claudia Cooley and Audra Seay. My editor, Patti Townley-Covert, you are a master of encouragement and word wizardry. My proofreader, Arlene Jacobson Aab, who paid attention to the little things. Lastly, my creative genius and designer, Whitney Wolff. I am always amazed how you take a simple idea and create magic.

Prologue
Common Threads

There is an eerily bleak sameness to the stories that have emerged from the smoke and ash of the modern day Armageddon in the hills above Chico, California. This is not a story about sameness. This is a story about difference…the difference that the Feather River Hospital family of employees made in the lives of their patients, their community and, most specifically, how four nurses stood hand-in-hand and faced down fire and fear. This is their story.

Here in this bucolic enclave, two lanes give way to three, then slenderize again, meandering through town. Towering forests reach skyward and homes peak from beneath pine boughs like children playing hide and seek. It's the predictably gentle lifestyle that draws folks to this little town. For them, its simple, its personal, and its Paradise.

Mornings come early for those who count themselves blessed enough to serve the community at Feather River Hospital. It's Thursday and Surgical Unit Nurse Manager Jeff Roach rolls out of bed a little later than usual. He's going to need perfectly timed traffic lights if he's going to make the shift change on time. Chelsea West, an Emergency Room Nurse, is already at the hospital with the RN House Supervisor, Sarah McCain. Shift change is under way. It is a bit past 6:45 AM.

By 7:00 the sun is up and resembles an overly ripe orange. Talk of a fire in neighboring Pulga is beginning to take on increasing importance. Within fifteen minutes, the entire sky first blushes then turns crimson. A small building on campus has ignited. Thick, black smoke and blazing embers the size of dinner plates begin floating across the campus and the Disaster Team quickly assembles in the conference room. When 911 calls go unanswered, it is readily apparently that hospital personnel are in full control of their own destiny. Charge Nurse Renee Souza and Unit Secretary Cathy Gaylord compile a full patient list. ER/ICU nurse Cassie LeRossignol arrives. It is 8:10, Code Black, and all hands are now on deck.

Beginning on the surgical unit and racing through each department, the men and women of this medical family meld. Cooks, housekeepers, maintenance engineers, and health care providers forge seamlessly into one unit with a laser focused mission: Save lives. Personnel quickly fan out. Sixty-seven patients are assessed, stabilized, and readied for evacuation. In beds and wheelchairs, on stretchers and gurneys, and ambulatory with assistance, frightened patients are moved to a staging area in the long hall outside the emergency room. A second facility sweep is completed, then one last check, taping each door as they leave, indicating an all clear.

Downstairs, the lights begin to flicker and the halls go dark. Outside, acrid choking black smoke obscures the sun. Employees pull their cars to the emergency room door. Ed Beltran, a retired Navy Seal and Emergency Room Charge Nurse, skillfully directs transporters and patients outside where they are gingerly transferred into private vehicles which are filled to capacity. The hospital has been emptied in under an hour. It's 9:00 AM

Cassie and Chelsea move quickly up the road to Cassie's car and notice Jeff and Sarah running toward them. They all jump in. Several agonizing minutes pass and the traffic has not moved. Thinking they might have a better chance on foot, they exit the car and begin to walk, instantly realizing their decision is pointless and perilous. They pound on the window of a car, stuffed to the roof with personal belongings. The single occupant stares blankly at them through his sooty windshield, ignoring their plea. An elderly man and woman several cars back let them in. The car doors and windows are scalding hot and the air in the car stifling. They are going nowhere. Clasping hands, they promise not to let go of one another, no matter what.

Again, they exit the car, this time running......stumbling...coughing...hand in hand. Sarah can hold her scream no longer. "I want to see my babies!" she roars at the fire.

Three cars back, a bulldozer idles. All four scramble up and in, turning the large metal behemoth into a can of nurse sardines in the passenger seat. The dozer driver has a two-way radio that squelches and sputters report, none of them good. For the first time, Jeff feels doomed. "I am not going to die like this!"

The smoke and ash outside their windows have turned day into night. Running again, they scramble into the patrol car of Officer Aaron Parmley, Jeff in front and the three girls in the back. They are surrounded. With the strongest cell phone signal, Jeff's phone is passed from one to another as each makes a final, gut wrenching goodbye call home.

Turning right on Pearson Road…an abandoned car…another on fire…and CHP officer Nick Powell whose car is disabled…one moment standing in the open, the next inside the sheriff's car. Then an indescribably nauseating sound. Tick Tick Tick The patrol car gives in to the fight.

Life and death. Every day, nurses choose by profession to face, then fend off, the reality of the inevitable. Yet they soldier on, embracing the brevity, the sacredness, the sweet gift of every moment. How was it that this fiery infernal monster was about to take their lives, forever extinguishing the joy of those left behind to grieve such loss?

So, they run…six people into the darkness of daylight. Officer Nick Powell grabs Cassie's backpack from behind. He tells her to walk; her lungs will not bear the burden of swiftness. Chelsea begins to shed anything that might catch fire, throwing her purse, then her outer shirt.

"Get low!" Jeff yells.

Then, inexplicably, the thinnest ribbon of fresh air hovers above them and they breathe in the fleeting freshness.

A cracking sound from the left, most likely a falling tree, then headlights. Jeff jumps into the street, waving his arms at the approaching giant. A bulldozer followed by a fire engine part the flames. With all six aboard, the engine makes its way up Pentz road, back toward their hospital, their community, their Feather River Family.

Encircled by a more distant flame, it is strangely calm here. This is what they know, these four who refused to let go. People are huddled outside the Emergency Room, patients who were evacuated and had to turn back, others from the community who have come to help, a father and son handing out water…and new patients who need treatment.

With a portion of the hospital still on fire, a buddy system is devised. Two by two, teams go into the blackness of the hospital for supplies and emerge with food, water, medication, bandages, blankets and oxygen equipment.

On the hospital's life flight landing pad, patients are placed in a large circle on its perimeter. In the center, a make shift nursing station, central supply, and pharmacy. Those who need oxygen for smoke inhalation are placed in an air conditioned vehicle with an oxygen tank and masks.

There are no org charts or disaster manuals in that circle, no name badge identifiers. Instead, the common threads of instinct, wisdom, decency, human dignity and excellent training have wound themselves tightly around these amazing people this Thursday and held them together. And there are four nurses who took one others' hands and promised not to let go...ever.

Nearby, Enloe Hospital has opened its merciful arms. A safe haven in this firestorm, its hallways and rooms fill to overflowing with the wounded. The makeshift circle of hope on the life flight pad at Feather River has emptied, save for four nurses, one with an air cast on her broken foot. At Enloe, familiar faces greet them in the emergency room. Feather River and Enloe nurses have joined forces and now treat the ceaseless flow of broken, burned humanity. Like a symphony orchestra with countless years of combined medical experience, this is their stage and they give the performance of a lifetime.

In room twenty-seven, four nurses sit on gurneys in stunned disbelief. They have survived the unimaginable. Soot stained fingers woven together, they exchange glances and shake their heads. And for the briefest of moments, they are patients too...and they soothe their own wounded souls.

It's the next morning...the next day...the next week...the endless ache of what's next. We watch and listen in horror to what has happened. The goodness in us wails in silent scream as waves of photographs from the front lines blister our saddened, weary souls.

As Paradise wakes up, stands up and rises up, an uncompromised beacon of hope shines through the bleakness. Those whose lives you have knowingly touched are but a few in comparison to the hundreds of lives you have affected. You never forgot the promise you made to your community: to be light bearers of integrity, compassion, respect, and excellence.

In the face of unspeakable loss, your mission remains an unwavering standard bearer...Living God's love by inspiring health, wholeness, and hope.

The lives you have saved, and the untold number lost, will not be measured by a beginning nor an end. They will, instead, be lengthened by those with whom you have shared your own lives.

As testament, we will pick up those common threads and continue to weave into our own lives and into this community the strongest of all threads - compassion.

Let us measure our worth not in miles traveled or ladders climbed. Rather, let us look to those who, like the countless heroes we have seen in these stories, make this world a better place by having lived in it. Let us stand on the shoulders of that strength and reach for higher ground.

Paradise California Wildfires - November 2018
Stories shared from personal experience Feather River Hospital nurses
Arranged by Liz Dickinson, Chief Patient Care Executive
Written by Wendy Vandergrift

CONTENTS

INTRODUCTION
PLAYING THE HAND, I WAS DEALT
3
THE FRAMEWORK
THROUGHOUT HISTORY, IT'S ALL IN THE CARDS
11

LESSONS

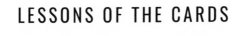

LESSONS OF THE CARDS

PLAYING THE HAND I WAS DEALT

Some things you just know! I always knew I'd become a nurse.

As a small child, living on the windswept prairies of the Dakotas, powerful family influence and storytelling forged my path to nursing. On my third birthday, an aunt gave me a toy nurse satchel complete with a white cap, stethoscope, pinch-on glasses and – joy of all joys – a "shot giver!" One toy does not create a specific destiny; however, the influence of strong women certainly created mine.

Courageous women willing to nurture my dreams and mentor me into my profession dealt me a winning hand. As you travel through the chapters of this book, I hope you'll reflect on the people who may have opened doors, paved pathways, and/or guided you through dark forests and back out into the light of your success. Reflecting on your journey can bring renewed passion for your career and your calling.

For some of us, the path was clear. With the exception of a few weeds, rocks, stickers, and mud, we moved easily in the direction of our goals. For others, the path has felt a lot more like climbing a mountain. We found the pathways extremely steep and narrow. In some places we could barely hold on to thin, crumbling granite cracks. Loans weren't approved, family circumstances forced us to drop out, a professor said we don't have "what it takes," or a dream job was given to someone else. Perhaps you're there now. Regardless, with perseverance, you can reach the goal of becoming a more effective healer, caregiver, and/or nurse.

Wherever your journey has taken you until now, I invite you to spend time reflecting on the challenges, choices, and changes that have created who you are today. Embrace the person you've become! Celebrate everything that is *right* and *good*.

While my story is a bit unorthodox, yours is equally unique. Reflection brings understanding and appreciation. Here's what I discovered as I examined my adventure into nursing.

Dealt an Inside Straight

Although my extended family set high expectations for their children, undoubtedly, the greatest influence in my educational journey was my Aunt Emma. Born in 1901, she embodied the perseverance of her immigrant family. Along with her younger sisters she completed high school, then teacher's school. Soon after, Aunt Emma left the Dakota prairies and ventured across country to the big city, Los Angeles, with her dream of becoming a nurse.

Throughout the first half of the twentieth century, nursing had a very negative stigma. Families were warned to not let their daughters become "those kinds of girls!" Apparently, the "oldest" female profession—that of attending to *all of men's needs*—and the nursing profession were considered to have many similarities.

On the strength of family values and service to others, Aunt Emma left home to pursue her dream. She graduated in 1929 as a Registered Nurse. Later she completed her baccalaureate and master's degrees. In an era when single women rarely traveled alone, she boarded a steam liner out of New York City bound for London.

While there, Aunt Emma attended missionary training, learning the language and culture of India where she'd been assigned a five-year tour of duty. Shortly thereafter, my aunt followed her "call to service" traveling by train, merchant ship, and camel caravan to a small hospital in Nuzvid. During her tenure there, she established a school of nursing and set standards for local and regional healthcare.

Over the next several decades she served not only in India, but also in Pakistan, Burma, and Africa. I first met my Aunt Emma when I was eight, and she was fifty-eight! A larger-than-life role model, she brought the world home to the prairies in her steamer trunks. Stories, legends, and dreams of far-away lands were planted deep in my heart. Although Aunt Emma was my strongest influencer toward a career in healthcare, there were other women who also cultivated my desires.

Emma's cousin Alma, also a registered nurse, served as a missionary to Egypt. She told stories of caring for the royal family in Addis Ababa. My heart thrilled at the prospect of adventure and caring for the needs of others in far-off places.

Then, there was Darlena, the lovely young nurse who married my favorite cousin Wayne. Darlena's uniform was crisp and white. Her white cap with the single black velvet stripe was simply marvelous. I adored everything about her uniform. Most of all, I was enamored by the navy wool cape complete with red satin lining and gold embroidered initials on the inner lapel. I watched with childhood envy as she donned her uniform and set off "for duty!"

At long last I attended my first day of nursing school. We nervously scanned the heap of books that represented so many lessons to learn! My heart beat faster as I was issued a name tag, small bandage scissors, and the blue pin-striped student uniform I would wear for the next four years. Real patients, real surgery, and the potential for developing real expertise in helping people regain their health. Could there be anything more noble or romantic?

After four years of diligence, perseverance, and grit; I was rewarded with a crisp white uniform, white hose, and thick-soled white lace-up shoes. Although the shoes were "flat ugly," my starched white nurse's cap with the full black stripe more than made up for them. How grand to recognize that my nurse's hat was the same style my aunt and cousins had worn. Recently, while going through a trunk in my mother's attic, I found Aunt Emma's cap. A note in her bold handwriting stated, "My Crowning Glory!"

Sadly, though I received my crowning glory, I didn't get the blue cape of my dreams. It was no longer part of a standard uniform. Ah, but doesn't change usually bring about both regret and promise? Capes and caps gave way to caps alone. Then those, too, were lost as scrubs came into vogue, but underneath it all—the heart of nursing and caring still persists.

Dealt a Full House

Nursing careers span a great variety of roles and responsibilities, and that's been true for mine. Working in a rural hospital complete with sixteen patient beds cultivated self-assurance and empathy in providing care to a very divergent population. Supporting a physician in the emergency or operating room or delivering babies were all part of my work in rural health. Being prepared for whomever rang the doorbell, night or day, built resilience and gave breadth to my fledgling career.

These rural lessons served me well as I transitioned to work in large university medical centers, community hospitals, and regional county hospitals. The teamwork, like that of a well-oiled machine, required in large hospital emergency departments taught me to respect the expertise of a variety of disciplines. From the moment paramedics called in, the emergency and trauma teams elevated to high alert. Physicians, respiratory therapists, lab, and x-ray personnel stood by along with nurses ready to do everything possible to save the life of a patient. Egos were set aside and we all worked together toward one goal—life instead of death. The results were often extraordinary.

Clinical experience provided a wealth of exposure to teamwork, disease and trauma management, and working within a system. All these lessons came together to equip me as a home health nurse. In the home, nurses practice in near isolation; occasionally speaking with a physician or advanced care provider. I became a patient advocate, educator, and healer. Expertise developed over a broad range of illnesses.

Home health required me to put together all my previous knowledge to care for people on the continuum of birth to death within the very community where I experience life. Unlike being in the hospital where patients lose so much of their identity, I observed patients experiencing everyday life—filled with their hopes, dreams, and suffering.

Laying My Cards on the Table

Throughout my career, I've been privileged to connect most closely with the role of educator and influencer of patients, staff, students, and leaders. As an invited guest lecturer at a large university hospital system in Hangzhou, China, I was honored to be part of a team of professionals that lectured to hundreds of nurse leaders and educators in two very large (more than two thousand beds) hospitals.

On the return flight, high above the blue Pacific, I experienced a couple of "Aha!" moments. First, nurses everywhere struggle with many of the same challenges. We want to "improve" (an oft-repeated word from my Chinese colleagues), and we want to make life better for our communities. Working with limited time, resources, and staffing are universal challenges.

Reflecting on the presentations made by our team raised some important questions. Did we have sufficient impact and was our information culturally relevant? Did what we shared, matter? Was it of value, and would it make a difference?

Goosebumps covered my arms as a simple thought struck me: "What would happen *if* just one nurse took one idea and put it into practice? More importantly, what *if* she shared that idea with one other nurse, a nurse I'd never meet. Then what *if*, just what *if*, that nurse took the one idea and shared it deep into western China, and *if* another nurse took that one idea into India or beyond?

The power of influence has vast consequences. It requires great responsibility. In a world continually in search of peace, perhaps nurses and health professionals hold the keys to a better future. In every hamlet and every city of this planet, mothers wish for better, safer, and healthier lives for their children. We, in the healing arts, have the ability to bring their dreams to fruition. Kings, presidents, and governments do not possess the same advantages that we do!

Over the years, great trust has been placed in my leadership skills. As a new graduate, I was hired to a charge nurse position. A few years later, I was invited to become the first paramedic training coordinator in our region, a job offered without my ever having instructed a single class. As a staff developer, I was allowed the freedom to create a leadership curriculum for an organization with more than fifteen thousand employees. The beauty of nursing is its malleability. With or without returning for an advanced degree, nursing allows us to easily switch up our career directions and work in a variety of healthcare fields.

Nursing gives us the ability to create our own future. Not only can we regularly restructure what we do, we can also blend and harmonize a career with parenthood or eldercare. Most importantly, we have been afforded the intimacy of providing care and connection to fellow humans who are enduring a season of suffering. When we practice mindful listening, we hear the stories of their lives, laments, and deepest concerns. We witness their suffering, healing, and/or endings—and that's a precious gift.

And sometimes in the process, we go in directions we never imagined—directions that help us discover things about ourselves. It seems odd to me that teaching is where I excel. My immigrant grandparents sent their daughters to become teachers. Eventually my strongest role model, Aunt Emma, became a nurse leader. And now, I find myself gaining the greatest joy through inspiring women, coaching nurse leaders, and consulting with others in the profession of health and healing.

What's in Your Hand?

Whether you're a nurse, physician, therapist, chaplain, or technician reconnecting to the heart of your calling is absolutely essential.

As we shuffle through a deck of cards, pay attention to card language, and learn a few card rules; ten secrets to ensuring success as a great nurse or healer emerge. Lesson 9, "Every Day Life Deals a New Hand" was shared in an address to matriculating pediatric new grads. Several weeks later that message was shared with an emergency department team. We added Lesson 1, "Rules Change: The Cards Don't;" Lesson 2,

"You Can't Cure Everyone; You Can Heal Many;" and Lesson 6, "A Poker Face Has Its Place." Audiences quickly and easily identified with the card analogies. Weeks later, staff, even those without a medical background, have reminded me of their favorite "lesson of the cards." The lessons are that memorable.

As you enjoy reading what follows, you'll discover the secrets to success and caring hidden within each lesson. You'll find your passion for providing care that goes to the root of human experience re-ignited or perhaps ignited for the first time. You'll discover tips for your success. You'll be provided with relevant and practical tools that can be applied to your career today. And, you'll read stories of real patients and real caregivers. Some names and places have been changed, of course. We all understand HIPPA, the privacy rule.

After you read and claim your favorite lessons, I encourage you to share that lesson with others. Add your own stories to personalize it. We become better when we share, remain open, and take life a little less seriously.

Life is a whole lot more like a game of cards than you might think. It's time to consider "how will you play the hand you've been dealt?"

THROUGHOUT HISTORY, IT'S ALL IN THE CARDS

"Sometimes you're doing really well, then, after three or four years, everything crashes like a house of cards and you have to rebuild it. It's not like you get to a point where you are all right for the rest of your life."

–Patti Smith

Card games and card language pervade our culture and provide glimpses into our own values and ways of connecting to others. Most of us have played some type of card game in our lifetime. Whether our first game was *Go Fish*, *Crazy 8's*, *War*, *Old Maid* or something more sophisticated like *UNO*, we easily recall playing it.

Children's games, *Old Maid* in particular, cause me to wonder at the subtle or not-so-subtle message they give children. Does a young girl receive the message that if she should fail to find her match, she will most certainly end up old, single, and repulsive? And what about young boys who easily learn the fun of *War*, where a bit of slapping around is perfectly normal?

Gender messaging to children starts early. Observe any small girl playing *Old Maid* and you will see "the look" that comes over her face when the spinster card finds its way into her hand. In my era, the *Old Maid* had a large, unattractive wart on her nose and a sinister look on her face. More recently the makers of the game have softened the tone of the card by creating a housekeeper *Old Maid* complete with uniform, mops, and dusting regalia. Is this an improvement or does it perhaps diminish the role of a person who performs these services in our hospitals?

Cards permeate our learning continuum. We create flash cards to learn colors, words, and mathematics in our preschool and elementary years. College students use cards to study for examinations. And many people use some type of playing card for social relaxation.

Card games are designed to test knowledge, skill, and wit. Some are used to entertain while others serve to teach wartime strategies. These innocent-looking, rigid pieces of paper have unwittingly been used to influence persons, cultures, and nations. Decks of cards have been used to create entire institutions of gambling and games of luck. These small pieces of paper stock have been blamed for bankruptcy, divorce, and yes, even murder. So how does something so ordinary, so ubiquitous, so innocent, become so nefarious?

The Name of the Game

The history of the playing card from ancient times to modern culture is both enlightening and fascinating. Card games are deemed to be the oldest, most long-standing game on our planet. According to Catherine Perry Hargrave in her book *A History of Playing Cards*, historians have established that the Chinese of the twelfth century were the first to have a version of cards for gaming purposes. In the thirteenth century, card games migrated eastward across continents, along with the trade of spices, following routes through India into Persia. Gypsies and fortune tellers who wandered throughout the region are credited with spreading games of chance. Ultimately, cards entered central Europe by way of the crusaders and knights.

During this time the very wealthy were the only people able to afford these beautifully handcrafted cards. Cards rapidly became a status symbol. Noting the great amount of money being spent on handmade cards, the Romans established a tax on these luxury items. The Ace of Spades became known as the Tax Card or Death Card. In fact, an Ace of Spades was the only card purchased, the rest of the cards were free.

Cards are played in a variety of ways with vastly differing sets of rules. Duels have been won or lost over them. Yet, there are essentially seven different ways cards are played.

1. Matching – cards are matched with each other (e.g., Concentration)

2. Tricks – includes a bidding process, suits, and trump (e.g., Hearts, Pinochle, Rook, Spades, Whist)

3. Rummy – drawing and discarding to form sets, sequences (e.g., Canasta, Gin Rummy)

4. Casino-style gambling – the "house" has the unfair advantage, but with some skill, strategy, and luck; there may be big wins (e.g., Black Jack, Poker)

5. Solitaire – single player card games (e.g., Spider Solitaire, Klondike)

6. Shedding – ridding oneself of all cards first (e.g., Hand and Foot, Mao, Snap, Patience)

7. Accumulating – garnering all of the cards (e.g., War, Fool's Paradise, Mille Bournes)

When we begin to look at the different type of card games as they apply to the work (healthcare) environment, we can find many parallels that evoke happiness or discomfort depending on our personal viewpoint.

When applied to life, these seven card strategies create some fascinating intersections, and some uncanny relationships come into focus.

Matching

While working in the field of healthcare or starting a new position, we usually learn to match or blend our style to that of our colleagues. Effective communication is enhanced by conforming to the style of those receiving the message. That's not manipulative; rather it is honoring their style.

When we need quick action, we may communicate in bullet points. Other folks need time to process and expect us to bring them the details. We learn to modulate our speech and activity to interact more fully with others. Connecting well to those who matter or have influence in the forward momentum of a career is a necessary competence for success.

Tricks

The art of using trick strategies in the workplace is paramount to creating great team partnerships. Interacting with team members, we bid for the work that we are best suited for. That allows everyone to function at their highest level. Declaring a trump happens when we are clear about our mission, and know the types of patients best served on our units. Following a suit is also a function of playing trick games. A team with clearly defined expectations and respect for its leadership has a great advantage in accomplishing the work for which they've been selected.

Most trick games require players to be paired. This necessitates partners to study, read, and respond to each other. Seasoned playing partners become adept at determining how to support and play off each other to the best advantage. In healthcare, we become valuable assets to our teammates by learning their strengths and determining what they most need to carry out their duties. Paying attention to these concerns helps us become mutually supportive in creating team synergy.

Rummy

Games of rummy strategically use other people's cards to enhance a player's advantage. While accumulating winning points, rummy players shed undesirable points as quickly as possible. In any career, there are those who are determined to grab the best position and score points with the boss, other colleagues, or friends, and they will often divest themselves of undesirable actions by foisting them off to someone else on their team. Though this may work in the short term, it undermines the overall functioning of the team.

When healthcare teams learn to play on the strengths of their colleagues and they cooperatively determine when to change strategies and shed unneeded points; our teamwork will be rewarded with a winning hand.

Casino-style

The thrill of casino games is associated with wagers and the risk of reward. In our work world, we may encounter associates who appear willing to take great risks for potential payoffs—whether financial or otherwise. Even healthcare organizations necessarily must take strategic risks in looking toward the future of medical care, reimbursement, and regulations.

Living on the roller coaster of rapid advances in healthcare treatments, while struggling with the frustrations of limited reimbursements, can take us through a range of emotions from exhilaration to alarm. Our emotional reactions to much of what we hear are based on the personal risks we are willing to take. And, as with any gamble, sometimes there are losers.

Solitaire

As its name implies, solitaire is a one-person game. Usually it's easy and fast-paced. The player may be required to practice concentration and/or patience. Cards may be face-up and/or face-down introducing an element of the unknown.

In healthcare, some practitioners work in near isolation. They may be researchers, laboratory technicians, or special project staff. While their interface with a team may be limited; their discoveries, analysis, and project implications may have a broad impact on the work of their colleagues.

Shedding

In these games, the goal of each player is to be the first to get rid of all his cards. This requires both strategy and skill. Keeping players engaged while deliberately removing cards from play is replicated in the healthcare world.

Years ago, hospitals were accused of doing "wallet biopsies," a term that was coined when emergency rooms took only patients who had insurance available to cover their visits. As a result, the Emergency Medical Treatment and Labor Act or anti-dumping laws were enacted. These laws require adequate patient health assessments and prevent hospitals from transferring patients to a lower level of care.

Accumulating

In this game, the player wants to hold all the cards. Holding the entire deck may be a sound strategy in some industries, but in healthcare it is counterproductive. With skyrocketing costs, marginal reimbursement rates, and limited resources both in human capital and equipment; it makes sense that hospitals should stop trying to do everything for everyone. Working collaboratively to ensure some hospitals are Stroke Centers of Excellence while others become Bariatric Centers of Excellence seems the best way to serve our communities.

By sharing our resources and focusing employee expertise, we can enhance outcomes throughout our communities. This will ensure we are good financial stewards of healthcare dollars.

When the Cards Have Spoken

The pervasive language of card games can be heard from politics to podium, from professor to pundit, and from practitioner to patient. Common expressions using card language reveal a deep influence in our daily lives. Card language can inform healthcare of its potential, its responsibilities, and its threats. In turn, it becomes applicable to interactions with our team, our community, and most importantly our patients. That understanding is central to how we play our hands. Consider these familiar terms:

- *She's been dealt a bad hand* —life can hand a patient some huge challenges that may not be fair

- *He's not playing with a full deck*—a distraction or inadequate knowledge can prevent an administrator from being fully present in an important situation.

- *Her life is a house of cards*—though a colleague may be holding things together for the moment, one more bad thing, unlucky event, or a new requirement, and everything will come tumbling down.

- *Wow, he got the luck of the draw*—through no strategy on his part, a colleague may suddenly become very lucky, and that can produce a bit of envy in coworkers.

- *It's all in the cards*—fate is supreme. The patient believes she has very little control or ability to change a future course.

- *Read 'em and weep*—before delivering challenging news, a healthcare professional had better look at his "hand" and be prepared for a difficult conversation.

- *It will come back in spades*—the effort healthcare workers put into their jobs will be recognized and rewarded abundantly in the future.

- *She is a wild card*—this administrator may say something or do something that could be embarrassing and beyond your ability to control.

- *He got lost in the shuffle*—somehow during the decision-making process, everyone forgot about the patient.

Although these sayings are often shared with humor or kindly intent, it is well to remember, "many a truth is said in jest." Whether it's patients, colleagues, or administrators—these expressions fit a multitude of scenarios for healthcare professionals. Beware, sometimes they may even be said about us.

RULES CHANGE: THE CARDS DON'T

Connecting to the Heart of Caring in a Rapidly Changing World

Some people with awful cards can be successful because of how they deal with the tragedies they're handed, and that seems courageous to me!

Judith Guest

Healthcare professionals, who have been in their careers for any length of time, certainly recognize the perpetual change of rules. We have become familiar with the mantra: "What is old is new and what is new is old!" The very cyclical nature of change becomes confusing.

Whose Deal is It Anyway?

Multifold change patterns have often been linked to employee fatigue, burn-out, and even medical error. Healthcare professionals are doing more and more complex processes. We're accountable to ever-increasing waves of requirements, regulations, and reports. And, we're subjected to never-ending scrutiny, yet are told that we must become the most efficient, kind, long-suffering workforce in the history of healthcare.

Once, simply being a nurse or a doctor ensured a mantle of respect and a cloak of trust. Now, we are told that our guests, a.k.a. patients, expect world-class treatment. Consultants tell us that our patients and clients are comparing us to Ritz-Carlton, Nordstrom, and Disney! Yet there is a vast dichotomy between my expectations of going to Disneyland for a few days and what I expect when I'm in dire need of healthcare. First, I really want to go to Disney. Second, I really do *not* want to go to the hospital.

When folks need hospitalization they are frightened, riddled with anxiety, and likely in severe pain. Our patients are longing for empathy, understanding, and symptom relief. Our staff is needing to be effective and efficient. We must work hard and fast. The dilemma is compounded because hospital beds are already filled with very sick patients; throughput stops. Emergency departments end up "holding" patients for days, just waiting for an open inpatient bed. Emergency gurneys are uncomfortable, curtains become walls, privacy and rest are non-existent. This certainly does not create a feeling of hospitality.

Yet, hospitals are held hostage with patient satisfaction scores. Like other service-sector satisfaction scores, an "always" is the only mark that matters. The scores are tied to reimbursement levels from payors, especially Medicare and Medicaid. Hospitals are struggling to enhance patient satisfaction scores. Currently, they are using a variety of strategies from the banking, hotel, and restaurant industries. Patient satisfaction scores reflect personal perceptions of kindness and caring. When healthcare providers are empathetic, listen attentively, and are genuinely "nice;" scores improve.

We truly want to excel in providing the best possible care, in a manner that supports the safety and trust of our patients and their families. In addition, we want to honor our employer and follow regulations. But it seems the more we hurry, the more we tighten productivity, the more we script our words; the less time we have for that which caused most of us to join our profession in the first place—to be present in a substantive way for our patients. Bottom line—making a difference!

This dilemma isn't entirely new for the healthcare team. Yet in this age of assessing, measuring, documenting, planning, implementing, and keeping up with evidence-based standards—the ability to spend time with our patients, hear their laments, be in service or in the present moment with them seems tenuous at best.

In addition, we are attempting to remain keenly aware of the nuances of our team, supporting coworkers and cross-monitoring them to ensure excellent communication while enhancing trust and honoring their strengths. Seeing team members in the best light is also known as giving others an "A."

Above everything, we want to enjoy our work! We want to love what we do and long for the opportunity to perform at our best. We give our jobs the best 36-40 hours of our week and grab the scraps that are left to offer our families. That leaves precious little time for ourselves.

Yet it can feel very wrong to let go of familiar work patterns. Getting everyone on board to let go of the old ways, so they can embrace enhanced workflow, is a challenge facing every administrator and front-line leader.

Whatever Happened to Time-Honored Rules and Traditions?

A deck of cards can bring perspective to the situations we face with new change patterns that appear ready to crush us. First let's look at how card games are played, and then we'll see how card games directly relate to healthcare. In a standard deck of cards, there is a great deal of consistency and sameness.

There are always 52 cards in a deck. Should a card be missing, the entire deck must be tossed. The cards in a playing deck are printed in only two colors —black and red. That's it! There are always four suits in a deck—Hearts, Clubs, Spades and Diamonds. Each suit has 13 cards and includes the "face" cards—King, Queen, Jack followed by number cards in declining order from number 10 to number one. This last card is commonly called the Ace. As basic as this sounds, it is important that you really connect to this message. For the thousands of games played with a deck of cards—that's all there is! Basic, uncomplicated, simple, easy to understand--so why are card rules so challenging?

Here's a true confession—I'm not a poker player. My face reveals way too much. Plus, I find the rules to that game complicated and confusing. Whenever I've watched or tried to participate, the nuances make me a bit crazy. The dealer calls the games, then declares how that particular game will be played. Numerous books have been written to help people learn, but alas, it is all still too daunting for me.

I enjoy playing *Hand and Foot* but find, once again, the rules need to be negotiated before even dealing the cards. Most of my friends say the host home gets to set the rules. How can this be so confusing, I ask? There are only 52 cards, two colors and four suits. No doubt you can add your own set of confusing card game rules to this list. *Bids*, *Counts*, and *Tricks*, are all based upon a complex set of rules.

With healthcare, the rules of the game and even the rules of the *house* or hospital change constantly. Time-honored traditions no longer exist. If you've recently changed to a new employer, switched from a rural hospital to a university medical center, private to public, not-for-profit to a for-profit, in-patient to out-patient, urgent care to emergent care center, behavioral health to public health—there's no choice but to learn their particular house rules.

And regulatory agencies make it even tougher. The Center for Medicare and Medicaid Services (CMS), The Joint Commission (TJC) and other regulatory bodies create and publish entire manuals to clarify *their rules*. Other game changers include the populations you serve. Although your license indicates that you are a nurse, therapist, physician, or other practitioner—being competent in the health community you serve is essential.

As an example, the knowledge and skill requirements between adult vs. pediatric practice is huge. Complicate all this with the varying department specific rules—think OR-ED-ICU-NICU-GI lab or disease-specific like oncology, respiratory, nephrology, and trauma. Overlay this with inpatient care, ambulatory care, and community health. Is it any wonder, healthcare professionals are as confused about how to play the game as I am about poker?

Who Changed the Rules?

Reflecting on the never-ending changes in healthcare makes it easy to take a dim view of the current situation and perhaps even indulge in a bit of nostalgia for the "olden days!" Perhaps you remember those days—those days before electronic medical records (EMR) when a health-care professional could simply jot a few notes on a flow sheet and hand-write a bit about the patient?

Recently, after being an invited guest physician to China, my cousin reminded me of the "chart" our family doctor maintained on each of his patients in the 1950s. A single line contained the date, diagnosis, and treatment administered. During his trip, my cousin once again saw this simplicity as each patient carried their own small black book in which their Chinese doctor jotted down this info.

Monumental strides are currently being taken in China to embrace Western medicine. Yet I wonder if this is best for their nation and what the cost will be to traditional Chinese medicine? Is the EMR providing more or less in human interaction, continuity of care, or enhancing trust?

As we reflect on changes in healthcare and healthcare practice, although not always easy or comfortable; they have certainly brought us a long way. In the early '70s, nurses were taught how to sharpen and reuse a hypodermic needle "just in case" the newly acquired single use syringes were out of stock! A colleague remembers adding a small morphine tablet to a syringe, drawing up a specified amount of normal saline, swirling to ensure all particles were dissolved, doing complex math for age/weight/dose, discarding the extra and finally administering this concoction by injection to her patient.

When I was a new graduate with a baccalaureate of science in nursing (BSN), I was assigned as a night charge nurse on a medical-surgical unit in a large hospital. Our unit had 26 post-surgical patients. The team consisted of a Licensed Vocational Nurse who gave injectable and oral pain medication as needed. There were two nurse aids who assisted with patient care. We cared for some very sick folks. At that time, cholecystectomy or gallbladder patients were in the hospital a minimum of five days following surgery. They had Jackson-Pratt drains coming from their large incisions and were in a great deal of pain.

Our practice was to put paper tape on the glass intravenous (IV) bottles. We drew lines on the paper tape to indicate the amount of fluid to infuse per hour. Then we visually counted the drops in fifteen-second increments, multiplied by four and determined if the rate equaled cc/hr. There were no inline devices to monitor or slow gravity feed; only a roller thumb clamp. The nurse aids were our lifeline. They would tell us which patients were ahead or behind on their IV fluids. My colleagues remember being convinced that we gave our patients great care. Yet, understanding current nurse-to-patient ratios whereby a nurse only cares for two to five patients makes me fearful that perhaps we left many things undone.

Another time I remember finishing a night shift, handing the keys to the narcotic drawer to the oncoming charge nurse, driving home, and crawling into my warm bed. The shrill tone of the phone broke my reverie. It was the day charge nurse calling to ask what time I had hung the liter bottle for the patient in room 6 bed A. I responded that I had hung it just prior to shift report at 0630. She gasped: "Well it's 8 o'clock, and it's empty!"

Most of us have probably experienced that sinking feeling when something unexpected happens and suddenly our careers and everything we've worked hard for just blasts us in the gut. My mind whirled with the ramifications of fluid overload. Did I just do harm? Did I put this patient into congestive heart failure or worse?

The day charge nurse and I discussed how the patient had been asleep when I changed IV bottles. Apparently, he had stretched his arm for comfort thereby changing the venous flow and suddenly gravity worked exceptionally well. Together the day nurse and I reviewed the chart of a 27-year-old male, excellent health, no cardiac condition, in hospital for broken femur—all good news. The charge nurse called the physician to report the potential problem. The patient was monitored without negative outcome. Whew!

Where's the Wildcards?

That had been a terrifying day, but others incidents made me as happy as being dealt a joker! The day we got the microdrip inline controller which metered a drop for every cc/hour--that was a godsend. The advent of the metriset in which to put our antibiotics, admixed by the RN and titrated to ensure the compatibility and flow of fluids. And, finally the day came when I was introduced to the new IV pumps our hospital was purchasing. That pump included a library of medications and appropriate dosing based on patient weight and normal parameters, presets for rates, and an alarm for every conceivable incident—it even had a KVO (keep vein open) feature that would never let the "IV run dry!" I nearly jumped with joy. While nostalgia has its moments, change has its benefits.

Many improvements in healthcare delivery, tools of the trade, and improved methods have given healthcare workers and their patients tremendous advantages. My husband recently had a cholecystectomy (gallbladder removal) in the morning, took a walk in the evening, and went to work the next day! I thought: *Well, if ever I have a serious illness, this decade certainly offers hope.* Together, we have made amazing strides in so many areas of healthcare.

Much of the rule changing in healthcare has been brought about by a deeper understanding of what we all can do to create more positive, safe outcomes for our patients and their families. So, while understanding *how to play our hand* requires patience and consideration on our part; playing by the rules benefits everyone.

As with the deck of cards, the one constant in healthcare—that has never—nor will ever change is the patients themselves. Like the 52 cards, two colors, and four suits of constancy; patients are no different than they were 25 or 50 years ago. Most Americans have been raised to be self-sufficient, to not need others, and to go it on their own. In addition Americans, except for those trained in healthcare, have limited understanding of their own health and the way their bodies function.

There are several reasons why. First, our educational system has had a limited focus on health. Though this could be changing with grammar schools starting to focus on nutrition, health classes typically have been taught when children are in middle school. Unfortunately, that's also a time when preteens find their bodies doing strange and unusual things. Too shy to ask questions, many students pretend to understand everything, especially when it comes to their bodies. Some teachers are as uncomfortable with this topic as their students! So, unless a person chooses the health field as a career, general education doesn't effectively prepare them for important long-term health decisions.

An "Oh, Wow!" moment happens when we realize that most people treat their bodies like some people play *Black Jack*! Knowing we need to get to 21 to win, we gamble that the dealer will bust, and the house will lose. Putting our money down, we place our bets on the table. Then, we cross our fingers and hope the dealer gives us winning cards.

Professional players understand many nuances of the game. They know their options. After seeing the first round of cards, professionals decide to hold, split, take a hit, or double down. Some pros are experts at managing the odds by counting cards or casing the deck.

However, most folks are not professionals. We don't take the time to learn the nuances of the game. Instead we hope someone with more skill will mention when to hold, fold, or split. The novice hasn't learned the strategies that lead to winning. They may simply quit after getting a little ahead, then move over to the slot machines. It's easier there.

The slots used to be called "one-arm bandits" because at least one arm got a little exercise. Now, all it takes is one finger to poke the button.

Most adults think about their health in pretty much the same way. We don't want to worry about our bodies and learn what makes them function well. Rather we eat, drink, and exercise without thinking about consequences. All with the hopes that we'll be winners.

Over the years, healthcare providers have had minimal impact on the challenges of gaining support with patient self-accountability. We struggle to impress upon our patients the reasons why they should make lifestyle changes. An illness can truly be a "wakeup call"—a brief window of opportunity in which to make decisions to do things differently. However, most of our patients want a pill or potion to do the hard work for them. If we're honest, many of us are like our patients! Most people resist making changes or putting in the hard work necessary to form a new habit.

When illness or injury strikes, perhaps for the very first-time, people start to realize they are not in control of their body, much less their future. Suddenly, they face a situation they cannot "fix!" So, these individuals come to the healthcare community—in fear, anger or silence! They come, trusting that we will do our best for them.

A High-Stakes Game

Trust. In cards, it can mean life or death. According to the old westerns, many a deceased cowboy, who cheated at poker, could attest to that. In healthcare, trust is an everyday reality. If a patient can't trust those with the skill to heal his wounds or fight his diseases, he could die simply because he refused treatment.

Yet, in America, trust in many professions is being eroded year after year. Americans don't trust elected officials or the news media. They have witnessed mismanagement and betrayal by financial and legal advisors. They constantly hear about teachers and pastors who have betrayed the trust of those they serve in the worst possible ways.

The Gallup organization has monitored trust levels since 1999. In their document "Honesty/Ethics in Professions," Gallup Historical Trends reported that nurses hold the highest level of trust. With the exception of 2011 when first responders ranked number one, nurses steadfastly hold the position every year. Trust scores range between 73-85 percent with respondents reporting "very high" or "high." In addition, physicians are consistently in fourth position and pharmacists in fifth. This high-level of trust is remarkable considering the outcomes.

The Institute of Health's (IHI) 1991 hallmark report, "To Err is Human," indicated that nearly 100,000 people died unnecessarily in U.S. hospitals because of the "screw ups" and mistakes we make. For a bit of perspective, 100,000 people is equivalent to a fully loaded 737 falling out of the sky every other day! That begs the question: "If we knew an airplane crashed every other day, would we fly?"

The IHI report includes the droll warning that approximately ten times the number (nearly one million) left the hospital "less well off" than when they were admitted. Mistakes are not intentional. We do not injure our patients on purpose. Yet we all know folks who were in the hospital and got a wrong medication dose, fell while getting out of bed, got an infection in their bloodstream or surgical incision, or ended up with a decubitus ulcer.

In the early 2000s, the IHI repeated its assessment with grim results. The report found that the amount of people dying because of medical error had been vastly underestimated. Still patients continue to come for care—trusting that we will always put safety first, that we will do no harm, and that we will genuinely care about them. The question is why?

In part, it may be because hospitals, insurers, and care providers have agreed to new levels of transparency. Historical commitments have been made to reduce errors and share outcomes data, root cause analysis, and near misses. The public is being given access to reports of hospital outcomes, so they can make informed care decisions. People in the healthcare arena appear to be holding this honor sacred and recommitting to doing everything possible to first, "Do No Harm."

Still, considering that the deck was once stacked against them, the person willing to don one of our "lovely" (hear the sarcasm?) patient gowns, is a gift. Everyone knows that one-size-fits-all gown. It is usually blue or green and open down the back. It is designed to humiliate and control.

The person who puts on this hospital garment is saying: "I am a human enduring a season of suffering, and I'm desperate for help and understanding." By embracing this viewpoint, we can begin to see the patient gown as a badge of honor, trust, and respect. Healthcare professionals have the privilege to recognize someone in a moment of extreme need, most likely frightened, and perhaps confused. An individual who is likely in pain—physically, mentally, or spiritually.

That person trusts the healthcare staff to decipher results, be straight with them, support their decisions, and provide expertise. Finally, they look to us to intercede for them, advocate for their best interests, and mostly importantly—listen to the cries of their hearts! They look to us to hear the lament under their words, understand, and care for them through their pain.

A Losing Hand

After the mandatory two years on night shift in medical surgical units, I was promoted to the evening charge nurse position in a large, busy emergency department. The department was staffed with nurses, techs, and surgical residents who cared for our patient load. This was the mid-70s and the positions for emergency department physicians, EMTs, and paramedics were yet to be "invented." It was an early spring evening, and all was running smoothly.

Then, suddenly, the big back doors banged open and the ambulance attendants rushed in with four gurneys, each carrying an injured boy. Evidently one of these teens had absconded with his dad's Jeep and driven out of the city into the hills to chase wild donkeys. Perhaps it was their inexperience or maybe there were other factors, but whatever the reason the vehicle flipped upside down pinning all four boys underneath. Sadly, two were dead on arrival, and the other two were in critical condition.

The surgical teams—consisting of neurosurgeons, orthopedists, and general surgeons soon converged in our department. Decisions needed to be made and as the boys were minors, it was my duty as the charge nurse, to notify the parents. The sheriffs helped us retrieve addresses and phone numbers from the boys' wallets. Then, I called the families. Relatively young and unseasoned, I had little experience with such a grim task. Mustering my courage, I picked up the phone, and adopted my best professional demeanor.

When I asked a sleepy-voiced gentleman if he was the father of Bobby X., he said he needed to pass the phone to Bobby's mother. After validating her identity, I conveyed the necessity for her to drive safely, but quickly to our hospital. I could hear the denial and desperation in her voice. Almost as an afterthought she said, "Oh, you better call his dad, the number is 555-1234."

I dialed Bobby's father giving him the same urgent message, "come now." This same call was repeated with all of the families. If the boy was in critical condition, surgical consent was requested. If he was DOA, the message was only to get there as quickly as possible. As families arrived, the physicians met with them providing updates and getting permissions for surgeries or sharing the devastating news that their child had not survived.

When Bobby's family arrived, it was clear that there was a significant rift between the parents. After the doctor shared the news that Bobby had died, the mother sought comfort and shelter in the arms of the man she'd come with.

Bobby's father stood alone—grief-stricken, shoulders heaving with shuddering sobs. He stumbled against a wall to maintain his balance. While I continued to watch, it seemed this daddy grew smaller and smaller. Every fiber of my body screamed to go over and put comforting arms around him in an expression of human caring. But, I didn't. Instead, I stood there frozen watching it happen. I was too young and inexperienced to let my heart lead the way.

As I write this story, I am again choking down tears. My professional training required a 25-year-old nurse to *not* hug someone she didn't know. RN's were expected to maintain professional distance and control. That event happened nearly 40 years ago, yet I recall it with vivid detail. I did not honor my heart or my profession. I failed! I failed at the art of recognizing and touching human suffering.

A Hand Well-Played

Fast forward ten years. In addition to becoming a far more experienced nurse, I had also become a mother. Working in Home Health Care, I was assigned to work an eight-hour shift caring for a ten-year-old boy who had been diagnosed with brain cancer. I pulled up to a small house in a run-down section of town. The door was answered by a lovely Hispanic mother and two small girls. The house was neat, but their resources appeared very limited.

The mother introduced me to my patient, Mejo, an affectionate name for a young boy. His head was swathed in a large white bandage, his dark eyes peeped out underneath and were alert. IV fluids dripped into his left arm. His sisters were eager to tell me all about their brother, sharing a video of Mejo's performance in a children's church production the previous year.

Two weeks later, I was again assigned to care for Mejo. I arrived to find the home environment very changed. Today the house was filled with people. I was introduced to several family members before I ever reached the room of my little patient. This afternoon, he was non-responsive to medication or conversation. As the evening progressed, it became apparent that we were on "Holy Ground." The time was short for Mejo.

Spontaneously, the family gathered to create a long and continuous circle of hands out of Mejo's room, down the hall around the living room, and back again. As Mejo's breathing became more ragged, I watched this daddy crawl into his son's bed, scoop up the boy's frail body, and start to pray. With praise and gratitude he returned the life of his son to God, who had lent the sweet boy to his family for a short season.

This time, I stood alongside the grieving family and let my tears fall with theirs. This night I allowed my heart to be touched by simple expressions of humanity. This night I did things right.

Understanding that rules change but the cards do not, informs us that our patients want and expect us to use our hearts as much as we use our heads and hands. Our challenge is to remain open to the call to care, to bear witness to the human journey, and to remember that patients stay the same. John Wesley, a 18th century theologian's words continue to ring true:

> *Do all the good you can*
> *By all the means you can*
> *In all the ways you can*
> *In all the places you can*
> *At all the times you can*
> *To all the people you can*
> *As long as ever you can.*

YOU CAN'T CURE EVERYONE; YOU CAN HEAL MANY

Embracing Healing in the Midst of Suffering, Loss, and Death

Like fanning through a deck of cards, my mind flashes on the thousand chances, trivial to profound, that converged to recreate this place. Any arbitrary turning along the way and I would be elsewhere. I would be different. Where did the expression "a place in the sun" first come from? My rational thought process clings always to the idea of free will, random event, my blood however streams easily along the current of fate.

Frances Mayes

When people feel a threat to their health, they can be observed taking a variety of actions. Some rush immediately to the emergency department often without an obvious need. Others wait it out at home; even at the risk of their lives. Healthcare team members often label these people by saying such things as: "talk about being in denial," or "she's such a drug seeker," or "he wants a pill to fix everything," or "she certainly doesn't suffer in silence." None of these labels help. Instead they blind us to a deeper dilemma.

In the U.S., most individuals have been conditioned to expect ease and lack of discomfort. Maybe that's why Americans have been taught to not look directly at someone who is physically different—whether that person is an amputee, someone with a tremor disorder or maimed by injury, born with physical or mental challenges, or other disorders deemed socially undesirable. Young children have no problems pointing out or asking about differences. However, well-meaning adults shush their kids and instruct them that it is rude to look at or question another individual.

The speed with which a group of "invisible" people can be created is striking. Invisibility is, perhaps, the single most destructive thing people do to one another. Not only is it perpetrated on those with physical and mental differences, but also on the homeless and elderly. Marginalizing others initiates a catastrophic slide into indifference and ultimately hate.

Through the Eyes of a Child

When my children were very young, my elderly uncle experienced an acute cerebral vascular accident or stroke. This left him with expressive aphasia (the inability to speak clearly), the inability to use his right hand, and the ability to walk. Our family loved Uncle Sam and included him in as many activities as possible. He adored my children and tried desperately to talk with them.

One day when my family gathered at an aunt's home for lunch, we brought Uncle Sam over to join our gathering. My cousin, Jeff, who was recovering from a broken leg and was now hobbling around on crutches joined us. As we drove home my six-year-old daughter asked, "Why does Jeff use crutches, and what is that white thing on his leg?"

I explained that Jeff's leg was broken, and the cast kept everything tightly in place until it healed. My daughter huffed with indignation and said, "Jeff's legs aren't broken. He can walk. Uncle Sam's legs are broken!" To my child, the word "broken" meant something didn't work anymore. Seeing through the eyes of innocent children reveals the perceptions and distortions we unfairly apply to those with physical and/or mental differences.

Studying a deck of cards can also provide insights into our perceptions of health—what it means to cure, what is normal, how we connect to those who are "different," and how we bring everyone into conversation. It also helps us understand that when we cannot cure or "fix" someone's illnesses or infirmities, healing may be possible. Though dictionaries might equate the two terms, "to heal" can be vastly different from "to cure." While people come to a doctor or the hospital to get cured, that is not always possible. However, what can be healed is found in the greater acceptance of a person's soul or spirit. Examining a few cards shows how.

The Jack Family

Flipping through a deck of cards exposes a few interesting characters. A unique characteristic was given to the Jack of Hearts and Jack of Spades—do you know what it is? Go ahead, get out your deck and shuffle through it, you've got time. Do you see it? They are called "one-eyed Jacks."

It's not clear why these two face cards are done in profile while all the rest of the face cards are in full portrait style. With the exception of these two Jacks, each face has been drawn showing two eyes. Though a person might speculate as to the reason, all the speculation in the world will never add that second eye to the two jacks.

If another eye was drawn on the card, that wouldn't really fix it. Those two jacks would still be different. This observation reminds us as healers to do everything in our power to relieve suffering and offer a cure. It also reminds us that when a fix or cure is beyond our control, we need to accept our limitations, recognize the pain of loss, and accept grieving as a personal release. It's impossible to cure everyone. When we deny our emotional investment in the inability to cure, when we do not grieve adequately, we lose the best part of us—our caring hearts.

People come to the doctor's office, the clinic, the emergency room, or a particular unit because they want to be "fixed." When an individual is suddenly faced with a real crisis of health, whether through sudden or chronic illness, a grave diagnosis or a traumatic injury, they find their illusions of control shattered. Perhaps for the first time in their lives, they are unable to "fix" things. Most adults have had the where-with-all to step in and fix their lives, their jobs, their finances, their kids; then with a snap of fate's fingers, it all seems to vanish and they're left with a one-eyed jack. When abrupt change happens, a person may find that everything he knows, the rules he's lived by, and the resources he's counted on are not going to work. And, that means something has to change.

A Mixed Bag

Members of the healing arts often find themselves both longing for and dreading change. Many seminars have been hosted in the name of "Change Management." Excellent books such as those by Eric Allenbaugh, William Bridges, Margaret Wheatley, and John Kotter among others, explore the topic of change theory. Gaining a perspective of human response to change allows us to be more understanding of the reactions we see in our patients

Regardless of all the available information, one thing remains the same: *change has no feelings*. It is people that give meaning and feeling to whatever change might be at hand. Change requires a great deal of energy, both physically and emotionally.

That's why most people choose to sit in the same chair at the dining room table. That's because it takes energy to think about sitting in a different chair. As energy beings, people are usually aware of the things, situations, or people that demand energy. So, if a person deems change as a positive event, it will most likely add positivity to that individual's energy bank. Someone else may assign change with negativity and for that individual, change will most likely drain and deplete her energy bank.

It has been said, "The only person who likes change is a baby with a wet diaper." Yet some babies actually don't enjoy that process!

Unexpected, unwanted change is most likely viewed as an unwelcome intruder. With negative emotions and energy attached to change, physical sensations often provide information that there is a threat or something to fear. When this happens, the human response is to attack or avoid the unwanted change. Thinking of the healthcare experience, few people interpret a trip to the emergency department as a positive change!

For example, if you have a patient who has just been in a motor vehicle accident—you will undoubtedly recognize the signs of fear and threat. Or, your patient may be a middle-aged business executive, normally in control of his empire. Suddenly he experiences acute chest pain and is on his way to the cardiovascular lab for stent placement. Again, you'll most likely observe a reaction to threat and fear.

> ## Unexpected or unwanted change =
> ## Threat + Fear = Attack + Avoid

Thinking through the framework of unwanted change, it is easy to see why many of our patients and their families move into an attack mode. Suddenly out of control, they are hot to attack anything or anyone who crosses a perceived boundary. Conversely a patient may turn toward the wall and refuse to talk with anyone. This is the avoidant aspect of threat and fear. Remembering the cycle perpetuated by unwanted change makes it easier to provide care and understanding to the patient without taking their reaction personally. It also equips healthcare professionals with the necessary tools to help families understand the reactions of their loved ones, who may be frightened.

Alternatively, let's look at a *change* situation that comes to someone who is in an embracing, open-minded, receptive mode. The change comes, and it is perceived as something that creates an opportunity or a challenge. The emotional response to this viewpoint leads to creativity and empowerment. This is a very different response than the previous scenario. From the patient's perspective, arriving at the positive aspects encompassed within change takes time and courage. For many folks, this acceptance never happens.

> ## Welcome or Embraced Change =
> ## Opportunity + Challenge = Creativity + Empowerment

Most individuals go through stages of grief and loss, as described by the work of Dr. Kubler-Ross, to finally reach acceptance. Children seem to have the ability to move through this change process more easily than adults. Younger children appear to accept what is happening and find the joy in their life regardless of the situation.

Once I had a pediatric patient, a young lad of twelve, with a rare condition that led to a severe lack of circulation. Eventually a surgeon had to amputate portions of each of his limbs. This boy channeled his creativity and passion into building miniature model cars and carefully painted them with a small brush held between his teeth. The cars were magnificent. He had a delightful optimistic attitude, and his room was a favorite stopping spot for all the nurses on the unit. With such an optimistic attitude, perhaps he grew up to be a wealthy entrepreneur or statesman. His charm, creativity, and empowerment knew no bounds and gave him a bright future.

The Jack Family demonstrates that there are many times I cannot *stack the deck* in my favor; nor could I stack it for that young boy. Some things simply are as they are. Yet, a healthcare professional has the opportunity to change her own perspective and understand the perspective of others. Individuals have a choice in how they choose to see their story.

The King Family

Like the uniqueness of the two one-eyed Jacks; there is also something unusual about the King of Hearts. Go ahead, check your deck, we'll wait!

Did you find it? Each of the Kings holds some type of dagger in their hand. In Diamonds, Spades, and Clubs, the dagger is held in the hand to the side of the shoulder. However, the King of Hearts has it plainly lifted and stuck into his head. For this reason, he is called the *Suicide King*. Again, there is no explanation as to why this card is drawn this way. Yet we can see parallels to the prevalence of depression and suicide within patient populations and local communities.

Studying the Kings, it is easy to overlook the small, yet significant, location of the dagger. When we provide healthcare to our communities, it is usually easier to diagnose the physical symptoms than mental maladies. Mental illness, suicidality, and depression can be hidden by our colleagues, the patient, and our communities. It is encouraging to see the recent efforts to remove the stigma of mental illness. The word "illness" implies that it is more than something strong-mindedness can overcome. When we begin to understand the many chemical factors that bathe our brains, we realize that psychosis is no more unusual than diabetes.

The King of Hearts also provides a lesson directed at all of us in the healthcare profession. Self-blame and guilt must be put into proper perspective. Often struggling with less than optimal outcomes, we frequently blame ourselves for not having recognized, offered, or intervened effectively. We hold ourselves accountable in areas completely beyond our control. We often perform a great deal of self-flagellation with the "woulda - coulda - shoulda" mantra. We all took an oath to help and not hurt, so we feel like we've let down our very profession.

At the same time, after many years in healthcare, I've come to realize, I am only human, and God has not given me the ability to see the future. My duty is to be of service to those along my path, to always provide care that is respectful, and to leave the rest to the divine.

Being honest with what we can and cannot cure is important. Healthcare professionals must openly share what is successful and what yet needs support. We must shed our "god complexes" and see ourselves as fellow journeyers within our communities. To be in service with others creates favorable circumstances to discover that which has yet to be recognized. Operating in isolation, or worse hoarding our knowledge, denies the greater health community opportunities to leverage our talents and strengths.

With all of healthcare's collective knowledge, medicines, and specialty services, it would seem that a cure for so many illnesses is just around the corner. When friends share a troubling diagnosis, I often remind them that the twenty-first century is a great time to have such a problem as healthcare has made (and continues making) incredible strides in so many areas. If a physician pronounced that a person was suffering from congestive heart failure or diabetes in the 1960s, the newly diagnosed patient would not have had many more months to live. In fact, chronic disease or chronicity did not exist prior to the sixties. People died of all sorts of things that are now quite treatable.

The dilemma nowadays lies with a treatment's exorbitant costs. We can manage a broad range of diseases and illnesses through costly treatments and pharmaceuticals. Yet, the same healthcare dollars could provide broad scope disease prevention strategies to millions. This conversation must start happening in open forums. What is talked about today comes to exist tomorrow. The future does not yet exist, except as it's called into being. It's in this spirit that Alice Morse Earle wrote:

Yesterday is history,

tomorrow a mystery

but today is a gift,

that is why it is called the PRESENT

The Dead Man's Hand

Cards also inform healthcare workers about life's fragility. Wild Bill Hickock, a famous Western outlaw, created a legend with his final hand of cards. He was killed in Deadwood, South Dakota holding a poker hand consisting of two black Aces and two black Eights; now commonly called the "*dead man's hand*" or "*aces over eights.*" Physicians and nurses alike must remember that sometimes an individual has been dealt such a hand and cannot be cured.

Though dictionaries define healing as a cure and cure as a healing—there are important nuances that need to be recognized. While most people hope for a cure, healing can have more to do with the mind and the spirit than with the body. One palliative care physician stands before her medical student class and declares, "100 percent of my patients die!"

After all the gasps and looks of shock and disbelief abate, she follows with: "And, yours will, too. Perhaps not on your watch, on this day, nor in this year, but we must understand there comes a time for endings in all human life!" Her candid approach is admirable. People in the western world seem obsessed with the notion of staying alive at all costs. While many cultures embrace and plan for endings, it is rare for Americans. We deny death, rarely talk about end-of-life issues, and are devastated when it's time to grieve the loss of life, whether it's our own impending death, our patient's, or that of a loved one. Worse, as healthcare professionals we often view death, not as the culmination of life, but as defeat.

In the movie, *Meet Joe Black,* a poignant emergency room scene unfolds in which Joe, representing death, chances to meet a frail elderly Jamaican woman. She looks at him cautiously, then asks: "You come-a take-a me to dat next-a-place?" Everyone must journey to that "next-a-place." No matter what a person's religion or creed, what that individual thinks is or isn't there, everyone goes to "dat next-a-place!"

It seems North Americans have sanitized the emotion and beautiful caring that go into bearing witness, sitting vigil, and honoring the journey of someone who is dying. Instead, it seems we're a society in denial; opting to place the ill or dying person alone in a hospital where others can take care of "it." In my experiences with home health, I've seen a great underutilization of hospice. A perception exists that if the patient accepts hospice, they are "giving up." Yet that is far from the truth. It may mean an individual has accepted quality of life over quantity. It may mean they are honoring a life well-lived. It most often means more peace, more intimacy, more comfort.

Making the Best of a Bad Hand

Healing comes with important conversations—fences are mended, love is reignited, moments are recaptured, songs and prayers may be sung. Extraordinary blessings often come when a healthcare worker stands on "Holy Ground" with his patients. Healing often takes place within these hallowed moments.

In her book, *Broken Open*, Elizabeth Lesser shares her story of living in a commune in the mid-sixties. Assigned mid-wife duties, she writes of "bearing witness to birth." Later she adds, "recently I find myself often bearing witness to death." Reflecting on her statement leads to the realization that never has there been a birth story from the baby's perspective—not ever. Either the mother, father, grandmother, physician, or nurse provides the story; never the baby!

An infant appears to have no knowledge of what he might meet on the other side of the birth canal. When that first mighty contraction came, what did he feel? How frightening was the descent into the birth canal? Then out he comes into bright lights, noise, and cold. Hopefully he will find familiar voices, warm blankets, and a new world of love. Yet we've never heard his story. Healthcare workers and parents; however, can bear witness to the event and share the story if the child wants to know his unique birth adventure.

Considering the untold infant version of birth; could the death experience be the same? Like the infant lacking sufficient language to describe his viewpoint, there's insufficient language to describe death's transition. No one has ever said what happens as an individual goes to "dat next-a-place!"

But what about the person who actually experiences the event? Clues can be taken from those who have had near-death experiences. However, these stories usually reflect the values and beliefs of the individual who has had the experience. Those who hold certain cultural or religious values frame the event within their own context. Bearing witness and providing comfort, love, and strength for the journey are all ways healthcare workers can alleviate fears and promote healing.

Inner peace comes when the patient is placed in the center of a caring experience. It does not come when we expect the patient to perform according to an "agenda" or to "understand a caregiver's work load." Healing comes in that magical few minutes when we sit and listen to our patient's stories.

Laying Your Cards on the Table

An admired professor, Dr. Wil Alexander, has done a great deal of work with listening to the lament of patients. He contends that *if* a physician would listen wholeheartedly to her patient for an entire two minutes, the patient would self-diagnose.

True listening isn't about coming up with the right answer. It isn't about figuring out what to say next; rather it's simply about being in the moment with no agenda—sitting with arms open, leaning forward, and focusing on what the other person is saying. That doesn't mean agreeing with them nor does it mean correcting their thought processes. It means respectfully listening to what they have to say. When the other person feels well-heard and well-listened to, then a more open and honest conversation takes place.

To be a mindful listener:

- Clear the clutter from your mind, first. Quiet your own chattering monkeys.

- Listen for understanding of the other person's perspective.

- Listen with your head and an open heart.

- Sit at eye level and lean forward. If standing, uncross arms and lean in.

- Focus on the words, inflections, tone, and body language.

- Listen for what is being said as well as what is not being said.

- Ask clarifying questions, or make reflective statements.

The current healthcare dilemma is greatly exaggerated by the many redundant, seemingly banal boxes we are required to click in the EMR. We are rapidly losing the art of therapeutic touching and listening. According to Zubin Damania, of ZDogg, MD fame, we are repeatedly faced with the moral injury and conflict of doing what is right for the patient vs. what is required by the organization, insurers, and government. This failure to connect meaningfully with others is what brings on burn out, accelerates hot tempers, and distances us from the very reason we joined our profession, namely, to help others.

By asking clarifying questions or making reflective statements, patients and their families will know a healthcare provider cares about their concerns. Enhanced interactions can be developed by using questions or comments such as:

"Am I hearing you correctly?"

"It sounds like that upsets you."

"Tell me more."

Drilling down without judgment and demonstrating genuine concern allows the other person to move from superficial to a deeper level of conversation. Often when another person is well-heard, they do not need our advice. The answer for their particular concern may even appear right in the middle of their own sentence.

When meeting someone for the first time; whether a stranger, casual acquaintance, or health professional, communication is often superficial and tentative. A new acquaintance may be assessing if we are trustworthy enough to hear their deeper truths. When a healthcare professional asks a patient a question, that individual *starts* by telling his story. It's easy to pick up on the first few symptoms mentioned. If we don't allow the patient to get to the middle or the end of their story, we may start creating a scenario or worse yet, a diagnosis based on our point of reference. Sadly, studies show that the average physician interrupts a patient somewhere around 20 seconds into a conversation. If that individual is interrupted during the *start* of her story, the healthcare professional may never hear the *heart* of an important message. The place where truth exists.

Listening with the best intent to another's story, makes it relatively easy to continue a conversation. If the person shares a viewpoint or misunderstands a healthcare concept—the professional can agreeably disagree without shutting down the conversation. Saying, "you are wrong!" insures that the conversation is over! A better strategy is to say, "thanks for sharing, it helps me understand where you are coming from. Are you open to another point of view?" With that level of respect, the other person will usually be open to hearing your viewpoint.

Though cure strategies often come through the practitioners, science, and diagnostics; healing is intricately entwined with the art of listening. Remembering to respect the *dead man's hand* allows us to accept the things we cannot change or fix, it softens loss, and dilutes the effects of emotional burnout.

Jokers and Wild Cards

These cards, Jokers and Wild Cards, are the most recent additions to the modern-day deck. In ancient times, kings were often entertained and distracted from unpleasantness by their joker. In healthcare, there are reasons to welcome light-heartedness and distraction from the pain and unpleasantness of hospitalization. The world can be a serious and dismal place, especially when someone is confined in a hospital bed. A nurse or therapist who brings rays of sunshine and humor into a room can make a tremendous difference.

I vividly remember wanting some humor during my maxofacial-oral surgery. After suffering with temporo-mandibular joint (TMJ) pain for many months, I went to the hospital for a fairly new procedure. At my husband Dan's request, the anesthesiologist relayed the risks of surgery. Afterward, I told Dan if I didn't wake up properly from anesthesia, he should divorce me and remarry. He replied, "the doctor told us this was minor surgery."

Not happy, I said: "Any time I am put under and am having my face half ripped off, awakening to my jaws being wired is nothing short of major!" Later my nurse stopped by to bring me a second tray of Chicken Ala King and chat. So much for "my last supper."

As the evening progressed, I chided myself for forgetting to bring along a good book. I scanned the wall magazine rack only to find a religious journal exploring near-death experiences. That rag couldn't face the wall soon enough.

This was no time for dark thoughts. About 10:00, I flipped through the limited channels on TV and, lo and behold—an exposé on near-death experiences. Was the universe trying to send me a personal message?

Morning finally arrived and with it, my sweet husband. A dear friend also showed up to see me off. No doubt, I was nervous.

While being wheeled back to my room after surgery, I wished for a joker to lighten up the place. I must have looked like I'd been smacked in the face by an eighteen-wheeler. Dan was pale and continuously patted my hand.

The fun didn't stop there. I stayed in the hospital for three days. It rapidly became apparent the staff of this unit didn't know much about caring for my type of surgery. Post surgically, I was admitted to the gynecological surgery unit instead of ICU. Their usual patients were hysterectomies and tubal ligations; not complex oral surgery patients.

The next morning, I buzzed for the nursing assistant to help me ambulate to the bathroom with an IV pole and suction in tow. There in the mirror I saw my face. It was enormous! With my jaws wired shut, I could only hiss out words. My assistant was ever so kind and attentive. I could see concern and pity pouring out of her eyes. While I sat on the "throne" relieving myself, she got busy filling a peri-bottle with warm water for a "final rinse!" This was standard procedure for her patients, but my surgery was on the face not the tush! I wanted to burst into laughter and say, "My dear, you are treating the wrong end!" Every time I recall this event, I giggle with delight. Humor makes everything feel a little bit better.

Some people are genuinely gifted with joy and laughter. Favorites with patients, their dispositions bring a feeling of springtime into the room. As important as it is to connect deeply with patients in their sadness or suffering, it is also essential to welcome opportunities for humor and happiness.

A current trend in American hospitals is to ensure that private rooms are the norm for patients. While most of us welcome this privacy, isolation and loneliness can be devastating to patients (often the elderly), who lack visitors and family. These patients try to pass their time and ease the loneliness with only a TV for company. During the misery of an illness— hospital dramas, the brutality of cop shows, or the scare tactics of evening news often accentuate loneliness, rather than alleviating it.

Hospital audio-visual services should be encouraged to add healing programming to their television line-up. Studies done by the folks at Planetree in conjunction with Mannheim demonstrate the positive outcomes of calming and meditative music accompanied by nature scenes. Light-hearted TV shows, such as "I Love Lucy" reruns, are also welcome. Laughter becomes an internal jogging exercise. Some hospitals are embracing television lineups that not only encourage laughter, but also demonstrate bed exercises, offer relaxation stations with instrumental music and nature scenes, and calming bedtime routines that prepare patients for restful sleep.

The value of jokers should never be underestimated in how they bring energy, brightness, and hope into challenging environments. The task of every joker; however, is to maintain humor that heals and never hurts.

Wild Cards also exist in healthcare. They are the rare folks who find something to distract us in the nastiest of situations. They thrive in the emergency rooms and lurk in other departments as well.

Dan was working as a paramedic with an ambulance company, the night he called. He was talking a mile a minute, and I could feel his energy pulse over the phone. Earlier in the day, he and his partner had been called by the local fire department to assist with transporting a patient. They arrived at the scene to find a homebound, very obese, lonely lady living in a filthy house. A kindly neighbor had been sliding a heated TV dinner through the door twice a day. The neighbor was going on vacation and was concerned about meal delivery for this lady. Going the extra mile, the neighbor had called the local fire department.

The day prior to the ambulance ride, several firemen had been to the house to assist the patient off the floor and up into a large, overstuffed chair. At the time, it appeared she had a broken arm, or dislocated shoulder; however, she adamantly refused to be transported to the local hospital.

Realizing the seriousness of the situation, the fire department contacted social services and together arranged a time to forcibly take this lady to the hospital. The ambulance crew arrived after social services and fire fighters were on scene. As the paramedics entered the back of the house, they were overwhelmed by the filth and stench. The metal white cupboards had long since gone pasty gray. The floor was littered with aluminum TV trays and trash was everywhere. One of the firefighters said, "Buddy you haven't seen anything yet."

Together the four men pulled the patient into a standing position. Suddenly it sounded like raindrops were sprinkling on their boots. *Maggots*! It was most definitely time to slap on a poker face!

Arriving at the emergency department, the paramedics requested the patient be placed in a private room. The paramedics informed the MD of the maggot "situation." The doctor gave them a skeptical look and proceeded to pull the patient's forearm down to start an IV. Hundreds of little maggots were around the edge of her inner arm fold and the really big ones were wiggling up tall in the center. For the first time, the patient must have felt something unusual, and appeared startled. The doc said firmly, "Hold still, we don't want to hurt any of the little critters!" This kind of wild card humor abounds in emergency rooms, and is one of the ways caregivers keep sane in strange situations.

Grandmother Swindoll, mother to the renowned speaker and author, Lucy Swindoll, is reported to have said, "A day is wasted unless at least once, you fall over in a heap of laughter." Researchers, such as professor Lee Berk, PhD, and the famous journalist, Norman Cousins, affirm the reality that laughter brings healing to the soul and to the body.

Jokers and wild cards remind healthcare professionals to use our gifts and talents to heal through caring and laughter. One-eyed Jacks, the Suicide King, and the Dead Man's Hand also help us understand that, although a cure may not be at hand, healing and wholeness can be created even in difficult circumstances.

EVERY CARD IS VALUABLE: A FULL DECK OF GIFTS

Valuing Each Team Member's Talents

A deck of cards is built like the purist of hierarchies—every card a master to those below it, a lackey to those above it.

Ely Culbertson

You cut the cellophane, slit open the seal, and pull out a fresh deck feeling the slick new finish on the cards—for many of us, it's kind of a thrill. Maybe that's because we're not often handed a fresh deck. Much of the time, games are played with worn-out cards.

New decks are generally *stacked* in a particular order. The top card has a full-sized Joker called the inspection card. It indicates that the deck was produced by an approved card maker. That's followed closely by the Ace of Spades, which is the tax card. The deck is then stacked with each of the four suits from Ace to King.

Incomplete decks are a source of frustration. So much so that most folks toss them into the trash. Likewise, in healthcare, it takes complete teams working together to deliver exceptional, high-quality patient care.

Yet after working as a caregiver over time, we may start to feel a bit worn out. And, opening a fresh deck and looking through fresh eyes can provide valuable insights.

Team Member Point Values

Each card has a particular worth as well as a place in the larger game. In certain games, some cards count, while others do not. In this style of a game, a player may want to throw out the twos, threes, and fours claiming "they just take up time and clutter your hand." Sadly, this same attitude pervades healthcare where the hierarchy of "importance" often prevails. Much deference is paid to physicians and nurse leaders while support personnel and housekeepers frequently remain undervalued or unrecognized.

Cheryl, a nurse in the Emergency Department (ED), experienced this unfortunate "power gradient." Prior to attending nursing school, she served as a unit secretary in the ED. She would introduce herself to each physician on the team and inform them that she was available to make their day run smoothly. Yet, a few of the physicians treated her disrespectfully. They refused to talk directly with her, didn't address her by name, and simply hollered out orders in her direction. This attitude angered her so much, she boldly told the offending physicians that she couldn't provide assistance until she was treated as a member of the team.

But what about the employee who doesn't feel empowered enough to demand respect? Cheryl tells of a patient who was admitted with limited information. Someone speculated that perhaps the admitting clerk might have more information on the patient, so a summons was put out to "ask the purple people!" Admission clerks wore purple scrub uniforms. Calling them "purple people" instead of learning their names and valuing them as important team members destroyed trust and collaboration. Like the 2s, 3s and 4s—some team members were valued, and others were *discarded*.

An Effective Opening Bid

Every card game requires good ongoing dialogue among all the players. Bridge partners, who want to win, must interact with some precision. Respectful communication is the essence of any high-functioning team.

Like some card games, healthcare is rife with acronyms, specialized vocabulary, and rapidly shouted orders. Communication flows from highly educated team members, many with postgraduate degrees, to entry-level workers with barely a high-school education. For many healthcare workers, English is a second language and that adds exponentially to the challenges.

Healthcare professionals live in a world of "thin-air commands." A team leader simply states that she needs something and expects "someone" to complete the task. That's like stating aloud, "my coffee cup is empty" and believing a good fairy will fill it.

It's no wonder that after many years, The Joint Commission's National Patient Safety Goals continue to list improving staff communication as a top priority. Communication is a life-long challenge. It requires every healthcare professional to continually strive for enhanced mastery. The way something is said, where it's said, to whom it's said, and when it's said—all make a difference. The words we choose to use, the barriers that impede us (e.g., talking through a curtain, with our back turned, or while distracted by a computer), can also affect an outcome. And, so does healthcare speak.

Understanding Terms

Every team has acronyms, but healthcare pros are deluged by them. Too often, not wanting to appear ignorant, we won't ask for clarification of vague terms and acronyms, opting to move forward with assumptions and hunches. And, that can be dangerous.

In a high-level committee meeting, a quality director started rattling on about something she called "HAPU." Boldly, a staff nurse asked the director to explain what the abbreviation meant. She rolled her eyes and curtly said, "Why, hospital acquired pressure ulcer." Taking it in stride, the staff nurse realized she had more experience in caring for pressure ulcers than the quality director.

Not understanding an acronym does not indicate a lack of knowledge about the subject. Looking around the table, it was clear that several other participants appreciated that the staff nurse had requested a definition.

Finding a Voice

Teaching customer service courses to a large group of hospital housekeepers affirmed that these quiet folks wordlessly spend hours cleaning up rooms and messes. Usually my classes are filled with lots of interaction and audience involvement, but this group of individuals seemed to find it challenging to give a verbal response.

At first, I thought it might be because English was their second language, making verbal bantering difficult. More recently I have come to understand that they are the folks who may have never been asked for "their opinion." From childhood throughout their school years, some people have been repeatedly told their opinion doesn't matter, so they should remain quiet. Perhaps because of this, patients often confide and share very important information with their housekeeper, lab assistant, or aide—especially if they share a common language or culture.

It's a mistake for nurses and physicians to overlook the role of a housekeeper or admissions clerk in the communication chain. They may be privy to key pieces of information that could significantly impact the patient's plan of care. As you can see, all team members are valuable! When team members are overlooked or worse, criticized, we lose so much that is important.

Another grave communication error is blaming or criticizing other departments for mistakes or delays. Such critical statements hurt the entire team, the healthcare facility, and the person who is placing blame on others. It looks and sounds somewhat like this, "I'm so sorry you have to lay on this gurney so long, but you know our lab!" Said with rolled eyes, in effect, this communicates: "You can trust me, but you can't trust our inefficient, uncaring lab." Doubt has now been placed in the patient's mind regarding their lab results. If they can't trust the lab, who else shouldn't they trust? At an even deeper level, they start wondering if they can trust the person who would say such a thing.

While it's imperative to communicate clearly with each team member, it becomes even more imperative to communicate clearly with patients and their families. As mentioned previously, patients trust the nurses and all those caring for them. Every encounter is an opportunity to earn "trust points." Trust is extremely fragile. It takes a great deal of effort to earn and very little to destroy. It is either being built up or torn down. Trust is never stagnant nor stabilized.

Trust is very much like the old fashioned "teeter-totter" in a park. It's wonderfully fun to play on with a trusted friend about the same size. Different sizes can be adjusted for by sitting in different positions on the board. However, when the much bigger neighborhood bully shows up and sits on the end of the board, he can hoist a child way up in the air. Then as he jumps off, trust flies away, making for a very hard landing.

It's much easier to create trust and keep it than to repair broken trust. Once lost it's almost impossible to regain.

Building trust with your colleagues can start by simply recognizing and introducing them in a positive light to your patient and her family. When it's time to change shifts or someone from another department comes to deliver a service, taking a moment to introduce them to a patient initiates a relationship. Saying positive words of intent to the patient, "You will really like Tom, he's one of our best therapists!" or, "I'm so glad you have Dr. Smith, she's one of our favorites," starts racking up the trust points. The best part is, others start living up to the levels of praise you give them. Soon Tom and Dr. Smith may well become your favorites.

A Hand Full of Hearts

Creating trust with patients starts by making small moments count. It starts when we clip our badges on and walk into the hospital or clinic. And, it can develop as we meet and greet everyone in our work day.

While wearing a badge, if a healthcare professional goes out of her way to be of service to others, people say, "Wow, she really cares!" Conversely, if a nurse is short-tempered, abrupt, a bit snappy, or otherwise not at her best, no one says, "Wow, poor Mary is obviously having a bad day!" Instead, that individual generalizes the observation and applies it to the organization, labeling the entire staff as being rude.

A simple acronym, CARING, can prevent that from happening.

Embracing its six simple steps can empower healthcare professionals with everything necessary for delivering respectful, kind, and affirming care to others. When we connect, acquire, respond, inform, offer next steps, and say goodbye—healthcare teams, hospitals, and patients benefit.

C = Connect.

In every encounter with patients, families, colleagues or customers; it is imperative to immediately make eye contact, smile purposefully and go out of the way to be friendly. To train its employees, Disney teaches them the 5/10 Rule as the preferred strategy to connect with guests. While healthcare is not Disney, it is an experience. Using this methodology, when ten feet from anyone, the healthcare worker is obligated to look that individual in the eye and acknowledge that he's been seen. At five feet, she must open her mouth and express something positive toward that guest.

Not hard, yet how many times have patients or family members stood at a nurse's station with no one willing to make eye contact; it's like aliens sucked every one of them into their computers.

While making rounds on a patient-care unit, Heather purposefully left her badge in her pocket. She hoped someone would ask her what her business was and why she was on their unit. After doing a couple laps, Heather met a gentleman pushing his IV pole to get a bit of exercise. They both noted that no one was looking at them. Laughing, Heather asked, "if we walked around here naked, do you think anyone would notice?" Their laughter actually caused a few people to take their eyes off their computer screens.

Perhaps the number of stethoscopes and paraphernalia around a person's neck pulls his head down so far, he can only see the carpet. Often a look of deep concentration and piety accompanies this action. Looking up, smiling, and being friendly can raise the outcome of patient satisfaction scores.

But actually, connecting is about more than seeing people. It's being nice. Nice counts. So does being friendly. Those traits show on our faces. And, patients definitely need our smiles!

A = Acquire.

Asking people why they are in the clinic or on the unit allows them to share their story. And, that helps healthcare practitioners acquire information.

Whatever your role, you can also let patients know that they, too, can acquire information. Requesting that they ask two or three questions during an exam, a visit, or shift empowers them. And, it allows you to know what's on their minds so you can allay their anxieties. Questions provide insight into the patient's need-to-know, concerns, fears, and even misperceptions.

The second half of acquiring is *really listening*. This skill requires being attentive, not distracted with the electronic medical record, giving meds, or even educating a trainee. Rather healthcare professionals should be in the present moment with their patients. Author Eric Allenbaugh calls it "listening with every bone in your body."

We'll call it the "Magic Two Minutes." Recall professor Wil Alexander's insights (mentioned previously) that if physicians listen attentively to their patients for two full minutes, patients will self-diagnose. Keep in mind that the beginning of the story may not be the gist of the story. Only hearing the beginning, then interrupting, can cause healthcare professionals to miss the real lament, the truth of the pain and complaint and the correct diagnosis.

Several studies have been conducted in which a physician made morning rounds on twenty hospitalized patients. In each room, the physician spent exactly two minutes. In the first ten rooms, the doctor stood at the end of the bed near the curtain or in the doorway and talked with the patient. In the following ten rooms, the physician pulled a chair near the head of the bed, sat down, leaned forward and spoke with the patient for exactly two minutes.

Several hours later the nurse rounded and asked each of these twenty patients if the doctor had been in and if so, for how long. In the first scenario, several patients couldn't recall the visit. Several said, "Yeah, he popped by" or "he stuck his head in" or "she was in a big hurry."

The most amazing results came in the last scenario where the physician sat with the patient. Every patient recalled the visit and said the time spent was at least five minutes, while some recalled it as "more than half an hour." Recently the study was repeated utilizing nursing rounds, and the results were similar. This connection for acquiring information is critical for providing good healthcare. Computers and tasks must never supersede listening attentively to our patients. Sitting down for at least two minutes is what patients deserve. And, so do you!

R = Respond.

Once the person you've connected with shares his story, it's now your obligation to respond appropriately. This takes a bit of emotional intelligence. The response may be to inquire more deeply or to reflect back what's been said to ensure you've heard correctly.

It's a gift to reflect appropriately what a patient might need—whether it be empathy, understanding, someone to commiserate with, or determining who can fix things. Reflection may sound like, "this seems very hard for you," or "this must seem frightening," or "I am sorry you're in pain." Responding also means sharing with the person what you will be doing for them.

It is important to avoid saying, "no problem!" We hear those words almost to a point of monotony. What those words imply is that "today you are in luck. Usually this is a huge problem." It is equally important to never say, "I can't help you," or "it's not my problem." Both of these responses rightfully irritate and anger patients. From a customer service standpoint, it's much appreciated when a healthcare professional listens to a patient's story and then says, "I can help you with that."

Responding well means being sensitive to a patient's feelings and fears. It's finding a quiet place for sorrow and bad news. It also means bringing the Joker to work to lighten a long convalescence. It is imperative to connect to the deeper feelings of patients, so we express our sorrow for their situation or cheer on their progress.

Healthcare providers need to advocate for a patient's needs. If someone calls because her meal tray is incorrect, fix it and do so without criticizing the food service team members. Responding appropriately means finding the time and space to connect to what others need. Remember the patient is never, ever, an interruption. They are the reason for our day.

I = Inform.

It's important to do everything possible to explain and to help. That means physically walking with people through the hospital maze instead of pointing to wall placards and giving vague directions. Informing means letting our patients, their friends, and family know what to expect next. Sharing what we are doing for them, explaining how long things will last, telling them when we will be back are all ways to inform our guests.

Introducing patients and their visitors to the people going in and out of their rooms is essential and so is informing them of the steps being taken related to a procedure, the rationale behind what's being done, and reasonable expectations.

Informing also includes patient education. First, don't drown them with information, people can only remember three or four concepts at one time. Second, handouts should be provided at the sixth-grade reading level. Besides providing handouts, patients need to know what's most important within that information—what they need to know and what they are expected to do once they are back home.

My experience as a patient led me to understand that a person sick enough to be in a hospital does not feel like reading or wrapping her mind around hard concepts. So, keep it simple, focus on what needs to be learned (without insulting an individual's current level of understanding), and keep it brief.

N = Next Steps.

Healthcare professionals need to look for every way possible to make things better—to make it easier to navigate the healthcare maze—to understand the unfamiliar terms—to know what to do next—to understand what will be happening with a procedure.

As a caregiver, you may be very comfortable with your work world, but our guests do not understand it; nor should they. It is up to each professional to be clear on what will happen next, what you will be doing for the patient, and what they will be expected to do for themselves. As a healthcare provider, you must accept that you cannot manage someone's disease process. Only the patient can do that. We must empower our patients through knowledge, tools, and simple explanations. Be clear about what, where, and how the next steps should be taken. Make sure they have a clear and simple roadmap to navigate and specific phone numbers and addresses for follow-up care.

G = Goodbyes.

In a world lacking some basic manners and kindnesses, saying "thank you" and "goodbye" or expressing gratitude, seems to be out-of-date. Yet, the airline industry always thanks people for flying with them. How much more should caregivers thank patients for their willingness to be poked, prodded, inserted, pulled out, tugged, hurt, cut, and sliced, among the many other humiliating tasks so nonchalantly performed?

Patients have a choice of which hospital or clinic to enter. It is every healthcare provider's responsibility to genuinely thank them for allowing us to provide our services. Simply saying, "Thank you Mrs. Smith for allowing me to perform your dressing change," or "Thank you Mr. Black for allowing me to do your surgery" makes patients feel valued. How might things change if at discharge a healthcare provider said: "Mrs. Jones, it has been my pleasure to provide you with care during your stay. Should you or your family need anything in the future, we hope you'll remember us and come back to Memorial Medical Center."

Getting back to our deck of cards and recognizing the importance of the entire deck, we must guard against self-importance or playing the *trump card* with patients or colleagues. By remembering that every card is valuable, every patient encounter important, and every staff communication essential; we gain trust and demonstrate caring. Ultimately that builds our relationships with others. Playing a trump card may be within our ability, yet it rarely serves as well as we might hope. Rather we want to keep the CARING acronym in mind.

C = Connect. Smile - be obviously friendly, and remember the 5/10 Rule.

A = Acquire. Ask great questions and really listen.

R = Respond. Find time and space to connect to another's need.

I = Inform. Share information, what you are doing, and how long it will take.

N = Next Steps. Always share what a patient should do next.

G = Goodbyes. Say thank you and bid a genuine farewell.

While playing bidding games and calling "trump" and "suits," Aces may be assigned as a "high" or "low" card, meaning they are worth ten points or one point. When an Ace is high, it exceeds a King. When an Ace is low, it is worth less than a two.

Healthcare professionals sometimes see themselves as the high Ace, the person with the knowledge to administer the healing arts to the suffering masses. By embracing this mindset, we arbitrarily place the person needing care as the low Ace, dependent upon our benevolence. That attitude means our perspective needs to change for in reality, the patient is the high Ace, and we are privileged to serve their needs. Without a sick individual who needs care—nurses, physicians, therapists, secretaries, and housekeepers would be out of work. Hospitals and clinics would be out of business.

Healthcare is about the team caring for the sick and injured. The Ace position also translates to our teams. All team members are important. It is important to respect each other and not assign high Ace values to certain team members while relegating others to low Ace values. A surgeon wouldn't be effective if she couldn't count on a sterile-processing tech to ensure instruments are ready to use. An ICU nurse couldn't do her job if a housekeeper wasn't ensuring infection control measures were met in cleaning an isolation room. And, if the medical billers and collectors didn't do their job, no one could count on a paycheck!

Just like a single card within a full deck—every employee, every patient, every practitioner is essential in the business of healthcare. And, when a team works together, there is great power in small numbers. Remember, a pair of twos, or three-of-a-kind can take a King or a Queen.

INTEGRITY: DETERMINE TO BE A GREAT PLAYER INSTEAD OF A CHEAT

Conducting your Practice with Honor in a High-Pressured Industry

I have always thought you could take the measure of a man by his sports manners—that is to say, the way in which he conducts himself on the playing field, or even over a game of chess or cards.

Graydon Carter

While playing cards, some people deal the deck, then play fair and square. They take the cards they're dealt and make the most of them, whether it's a winning or a losing hand. Other folks employ many devious strategies. They may stack the deck, switch the deck, hide cards up their sleeves or use sleight of hand. Players who cheat soon gain a bad reputation.

Although unsuspecting people continue to be taken advantage of by card sharks, good players try to avoid them. Cheats do not make great friends or colleagues. To be a great player or a cheat depends almost entirely on one's personal integrity.

The choice to have personal integrity is a deliberate moral decision, one that matters in healthcare. It doesn't simply "happen." You are either taught to have integrity or learn it from the school of hard knocks. Integrity means living by a strong internal moral compass. Yet in today's world, many folks seem to have missed this class. Integrity has become a commodity in short supply. It appears easier to do "what feels good" rather than do "what's right!" Integrity, however, is essential in healthcare. Using the most current information to provide treatment is the first step. The second step is to acknowledge and report when an error has been made. Many organizations currently exist to help healthcare institutions change outcomes by shedding light on what happens with "near misses" or what I call, "Oh Oops!" That's the internal feeling of fear mixed with relief when a healthcare professional knows he nearly made a mistake but caught himself before anything bad happened. This gut reaction should be an impetus to report what was happening that nearly caused the adverse event. The Institute for Safe Medication Practices continues to report that more than 1.5 million medication errors actually do occur annually. By learning from near mistakes, actionable steps can be taken to prevent more serious, life-threatening errors. Everyone would benefit if healthcare workers self-reported and stood in the gap as an advocate for patient safety.

To learn more about adverse events, avoidable harms, error by omission or commission, and "good catch programs," please visit the websites of these public agencies:

- The Agency for Healthcare Research and Quality

- The Institute of Medicine

- The Institute for Healthcare Improvement

- National Quality Forum

- Institute for Safe Medication Practices

According to Herbert William Heinrich in his book *Industrial Accident Prevention: A Scientific Approach*," printed in 1939, for every three hundred "near misses," 29 minor injuries and one major injury or serious harm results. We've had this data a very long time. This very old study should awaken the courage to self-report the times we have that "Oh Oops!" feeling. Most often error is not caused by negligence or deliberate action; rather it is a set of circumstances or processes that cause healthcare providers to be distracted, careless, overwhelmed, or otherwise stymied. By cultivating an environment where it is safe to be honest, such reporting could go a long way toward preventing errors.

Every time we engage in playing cards or working in healthcare, we have the choice to walk with integrity, be truthful with ourselves and others, and do the right thing at the right time for the right reason. In nursing, we're engrained with patient rights: right patient, right medication, right time, right dose, right route, right reaction, right documentation, and on and on. Yet for a wide variety of reasons, these basic rights are often jeopardized.

Our work loads are too heavy. We're being asked to do more with less. Things "fall off our plates" not because we wish to do harm, rather because our work plates overflow with responsibilities. Work piles up because we need excessive documentation, sometimes forcing us to care more for our computers than our patients.

We're increasingly responsible to measure more and more outcomes, yet we have access to less complete data. All said, it is imperative to become honest with that which we can do and balance those tasks against what is right to do.

Every day a healthcare professional puts on a uniform, lab coat, and badge and walks into work, that individual has to make the decision to walk with integrity. Some swore an oath by Hippocrates to "first do no harm." Others pledged by Nightingale to "abstain from whatever is deleterious or mischievous." Whatever their profession, healthcare workers have a code of conduct to uphold. Playing with integrity is clearly defined.

Truth is, sometimes this is easier said than done. Some days are much more challenging than others. At times, it's very tempting to cheat and cover up things that happen in hopes you won't get caught. You breathe a silent plea to the Creator that no harm will befall your patient. You fear, if you confess to error, you may lose your job. This pressure may even tempt you to *use sleight of hand* or tuck a *card up a sleeve*.

Healthcare professionals often hear the saying: "no harm, no foul." Yet without the integrity to identify "near misses," we ultimately become part of a system failure that will assuredly happen in the future. When a huge error occurs and we're secretly glad it's not ours, do we remember how many times we "nearly" made the same error? It's critical to decide now, today, how to handle difficult decisions. We can't do so in the moment if we haven't already committed to working with integrity.

Perhaps even more difficult than being self-accountable and re-sponsible is what happens when a trusted colleague asks us to "look the other way." When a breach or error that seems to have no negative conse-quence occurs, will we have the courage to speak up? How will we do the "right thing" when it is extremely uncomfortable to do so? Will we *bluff* or act with openness and candor? Or will we shove the card under the rug? Will we have the courage to *make the call* and report the incident, regard-less of putting a personal relationship in jeopardy?

During this challenging time, it's important to remember that being a *cheat* not only does a personal disservice, it creates an enormous breach of trust with patients. At those times we need to remember the trust patients put in those taking care of them. In a world full of disap-pointment fueled by stories of broken trust and greed, nurses and other complimentary healthcare providers continue to hold the highest levels of trust of any career group in America. Most patients are gracious with truthfulness. They want to hear the truth, even if a mistake has been made. Good intentions and honesty are often rewarded with enhanced trust by patients and other team members.

Some of the most valuable career lessons come directly from pa-tients. A pivotal story has informed many of my lectures to new hires and new graduates.

My weekend on call was going smoothly. I'd made all but one of my home health appointments to visit my patients. As I drove to that last appointment, I recalled what I already knew about the client. In the weekly case conference, I learned that this patient had been on our case list for several years, even though this was my first visit. I also remembered that he had many rounds of antibiotics but today, I was only changing a small bandage on his head. Other than that, I only knew he'd made an odd request: "Knock twice on the door. It will be open. Come on in and follow my voice to the back bedroom."

As a matter of practice, I connect with people as quickly and simply as possible by looking around their house and finding a common conversation item. So, on this particular day, I grabbed my nursing bag, knocked loudly on the door and heard Mark's voice summon me to the back. Scanning the living room, I noted rows of DVD's and video cassettes rivaling Blockbuster's. I had a snappy comment ready: "Next time I need to rent a movie, Mark, I'll come to your house!"

However, upon entering the room, I stopped short. Seasoned as I was, I was not prepared for Mark. It took every fiber of my being to not shudder. Rather, I slapped on my poker face. The flippant comment about renting movies evaporated. In front of me sat the most scarred, ruined, damaged person I'd ever seen. Only Mark's beautiful, deep brown eyes held me in check.

Mark had sustained burn damage over every part of his body. In addition, he had lost portions of all four limbs. Scanning the room quickly to pull myself back together, I saw a photograph of his parents. "No that won't do," I thought. But there it was, a picture of a stunning blond young lady. So, I said, "Mark, tell me about the beautiful blond!"

It was a story of tragedy and profound loss. The beautiful girl had been his fiancé. He told me of the delightful day they spent in the mountains, the drive home in the fog, the car careening over the side of the mountain, rolling several times and bursting into flames. His fiancé did not survive, and I wondered silently if Mark was sorry he had.

As I continued to dress and bandage Mark's wounds, we talked about his healthcare journey in my hospital. Suddenly, I looked at Mark and exclaimed, "Wow, you really know us! I bet you arrived on our helipad, were taken to our emergency department, then into surgery, ICU, medical units, and rehab."

"Oh yes, and orthopedics, too," he responded.

I continued, "I teach nurses and orient hospital staff every month, do you have a message I can share with them?"

"Yes, please tell them to always, *always*, listen to their patients!"

Evidently, Mark had made it through many critical days in the ICU burn unit and was now on our orthopedic unit. He had lost one leg immediately following the accident. His remaining leg had been badly injured, but surgery had been delayed until his other systems stabilized.

It was his second night post-op following the surgical repair for the crushed bones. Heavy pressure bandages had been placed over the surgical site. He was in traction and felt like he was doing as well as could be expected. The orthopedic resident had made evening rounds assuring Mark that the antibiotics were running as prescribed, and the pain level should be controlled.

However, Mark told me he awoke shortly after midnight with what he described as "horrific, infection pain!"

I stopped him right then. "Mark," I cried, "I have heard of searing, goring, boring, aching, and pressing elephants on the chest pain, but never infection pain. What do you mean by 'infection pain'?"

"When you've had as many infections as I have," he replied, "you immediately know the searing nature of the pain. So, I put on my call light and told a young nurse what was happening. She checked my temperature, which was about 100^0 F. So, she had me take deep breaths to prevent post-surgical pneumonia. Then she checked my antibiotics to make sure they were running at the right rate. She checked the pulse on my foot, my blood pressure, and of course, the surgical bandages. They looked fine. Then she said everything looked good and my pain medications weren't due for a couple more hours."

Mark recalled that during evening rounds, the resident had complained to the nurse that he'd been on for 36 hours. Exhausted he said: "Everything looks good. I'm going to bed, don't call me."

Still the night nurse called, and the resident abruptly shouted: "Call me back when his temperature is over 101^0!"

Mark's temperature never reached 101^0. The diligent nurse watched all night, hoping she had made the right decision. She did not call the resident again nor did she activate the chain of command. During morning rounds, the chief surgeon loudly berated the resident for his failure to personally respond to the call. Mark lost his leg. No one will ever know if the need to amputate was linked to the poor decisions on the night shift or one of many other complications.

So what steps might a more experienced nurse have taken? Recalling my early years in patient care, I can remember internally questioning my own clinical judgements. I'd start by asking myself if I could trust my knowledge and thought processes—in other words, could I trust my logic, my brain?

To this day, when I go shopping at Nordstrom's, I'll sometimes find an item that exceeds my budget, yet with a few mental gymnastics, I can easily convince myself that given that item's great benefits, it will easily pay for itself. So, logic is not always a good indicator. The inexperienced nurse reasoned according to what she knew, and that failed her.

Could going by the heart have made a difference? A caring heart may be wonderfully loving, but is also well-known for the way it can lead someone astray. And it could also incur the wrath of the resident who said "don't call me."

Yet gut instinct rarely fails. Over time I learned to intuitively listen to the deeper, quieter instinct that rarely leads to a wrong conclusion. Even our body language reflects when gut instinct should be trusted. Have you ever watched a seasoned practitioner cross his arms over his mid-section and lean over them, eyes closed, while agonizing with a decision? He's trusting his gut because he knows that will help him determine the best solution.

So how could the sleepy resident's response have been handled in a way that could have led to a different result? Seasoned nurses know they can always use the chain of command and call the attending. Still the exhausted resident needs to be kept in mind. Sometimes with acute lack of sleep, a resident may not be his most rationale self. Rather than be too hasty, the first option might be to encourage the nurse to call the resident one more time. He may not have fallen asleep as easily as he'd hoped. Perhaps he, too, was rethinking his decision.

The night nurse could call again and simply state: "I'm very uncomfortable with your decision, but I know you're tired. If you'd rather, I can call the chief physician." This gives a compassionate option that puts the decision in the resident's hands. Either he rethinks his course of action or someone else will. Many a resident is likely grateful for a wise nurse, who prevented a serious mistake.

Mark's lesson must never be forgotten. "Tell them to always, *al-*

ways listen to their patient!" Whether playing a game of cards or embroiled in the game of life, healthcare providers must determine whether to have the integrity to *make the call,* let something *slide,* or *cheat.* Critical decisions must be made in the quiet of our own hearts and minds.

CLAIM YOUR ACE

Building a Bank of Personal Skills and Confidence

When you are playing with a stacked deck, compete even harder. Show the world how much you will fight for the winner's circle. If you do, someday the cellophane will crackle off a fresh pack, one that belongs to you, and the cards will be stacked in your favor.

Pat Riley

Ace terminology abounds in American culture. People often say things like, "I aced my exam" or "she is an ace nurse." Great work is assigned the term "ace."

You're Number One

Looking at a deck of cards as related to healthcare professionals, the acronym ACE becomes a powerful mantra for self-acceptance.

A = *Authenticity* — the trueness and fidelity to your core values and destiny

C = *Creativity* — the talents and intuition that sets you apart from others

E = *Expertise* — the training and experience that leverage your advantage

Authenticity

Popeye famously said, "I yam what I yam, and that's all that I yam." This simplistic form of authenticity can teach healthcare professionals the value of being real or genuine. In an age of increasing pressure to conform to an unrealistic standard of beauty and excellence, it is a wonderful gift to simply relax and accept ourselves.

Trueness to an internal compass and personal calling are among the greatest assets in self-acceptance. Understanding and accepting that each individual (including you) is uniquely and divinely created unleashes the power to embrace a sense of purpose. Each person has a mission to fulfill—and that may be especially valid for us.

Fidelity to a unique purpose helps healthcare professionals understand that we were created for the task to which we were destined. Wisdom challenges us to accept ourselves as we are, not how we might wish we "would," "could" or "should" be. Seeing ourselves clearly makes it easier to administer to ourselves the large doses of grace we often give to others.

By being true to ourselves, we become less of an imposter or "poser." Life becomes unmanageable when we project a widely divergent image to colleagues, family, and maybe even our spouse. Every aspect of life becomes vastly more simplified when we stop telling or showing a different version of ourselves to others. That can be exhausting!

When asked what he did for a living, my cousin said, "I sell steel, and it suits me!" I'd never heard anyone describe themselves this way for the job they performed. How would our lives change if we start to focus on our unique suitability for our profession and remove from our thoughts wrong beliefs about ourselves?

Authenticity starts when we become truthful and accepting of who and what we are. It grows when we quit pretending and stop fibbing to ourselves and others. Being genuine becomes the reality when who you are and what you believe in—the core of your inner self—is exactly how you act, talk, and express yourself.

Phoniness is apparent even to very young children. Fake people make claims even they don't believe. They are simply *bluffing*!

A wise professor once posited this question to his class, "If in this life, you spend your time trying to be someone else, then who in this life, will be you?" Spending time reading and reflecting on your authenticity will help you embrace yourself. And, you have infinite worth!

Creativity

Imaginative artistry is a divine gift—one that distinguishes human beings from all other creatures on this planet. Though we all have creative ability—for many, the seeds of creativity have remained dormant just waiting to be watered.

As uniquely different as each individual life; so are the gifts of creativity each healthcare professional brings to the world, the workplace, and our patients. It's sad to hear people lament, "I am just not creative!" Perhaps they see creativity as only valuable if they are considered masters of a particular genre; like being an artist, a musician, or a street performer. Yet, as healthcare professionals we use creativity every single day to manage our responsibilities. Creativity fills us with positive energy. That's a lesson I learned firsthand.

Years ago, I was feeling overwhelmed with my job. My children were small, and my energy reservoir was depleted. I needed restoration. On a whim, I sent my husband and kids to the park and pulled out a grapevine wreath and the silk florals I'd purchased months earlier. As I started wiring and gluing the flowers, I suddenly became mindful that I was humming a happy tune. It had been a long time since I had done that. I vowed from that day forward to take regular, calendared dates with myself to enjoy places and projects that fill me with creativity and energy.

A vibrant life and good health depend on monitoring our energy levels. Some of you may want to shout: "You don't understand, I'm too busy to take care of myself!"

"Really? If you don't take care of your personal health and wellness, who will?" No one should apologize for taking an occasional day off work, simply to play. Folks who claim they are too valuable to their profession to take a vacation are only lying to themselves and putting their health and well-being at risk. Mounting evidence demonstrates that when we block our own energy, disease begins to form in our bodies.

Connecting to our creative selves not only restores us, but also allows us to become playful and light-hearted. It unleashes our ability to connect more fully with our patients. When our buckets are full, we can fill the buckets of others. When we run dry, we may be impatient, gruff, and out of sorts. This emotional state hurts everyone.

Creativity is all around us. Think of the many ways healthcare workers connect to their patients. Perhaps it's convincing a child to permit their blood pressure to be taken by giving their arm "a hug." Or maybe it's a complex medical procedure being framed into everyday language. Or figuring out how to splint a limb for maximal healing or performing a challenging surgical procedure.

Developing creativity enhances our ability to care for patients. Healthcare is a true blend of art and science. Honoring our gifts in such a way that they reflect creativity creates magical moments for patients and provides innovative solutions.

Expertise

The last letter in ACE reminds us how important it is to embrace and claim our competence. Each of us has specialized areas in which we bring valuable proficiency to our teams, patients and communities. Yet, when asked, "What do you do?" frequently our colleagues reply, "Oh, I'm just a nurse!"

There's no such thing as "just a nurse!" Nursing, like all of the healthcare professions, requires high-level skills, decision making, and emotional sensitivity. Each individual who has passed their boards has amassed an amazing amount of knowledge. Experience grows this base, and skill competence is perfected through repetition.

Anyone who has accrued ten thousand hours in a single endeavor can claim to be an expert in that area. Working full-time equals a bit more than two thousand hours per year. Hence, anyone with five years of experience in any area of the healthcare field can claim to be an expert.

Asking men and women what they do for a living provides a revealing distinction in gender response. Many men have a cool, quick commercial, also called an "elevator speech!" In a sentence or two they share their title and promote their line of work. Women, however, tend to be evasive, downplaying their role or minimizing it. They often reply, "Oh, I do lots of things. Mostly I'm a mom, but I also work as a dietitian, and I volunteer at school and—and—and!" Claiming your expertise requires us to sit quietly, spend time clarifying, and then practicing our "commercials" until repeating them becomes second nature.

Building ACE

Authenticity. Creativity. Expertise. As healthcare professionals, who want to grow in these areas, we need to learn and understand our basic temperament style, our leadership strengths, and our unique, personal edge. This knowledge starts building the appropriate terminology with which to accurately describe ourselves. Many websites and books offer valuable tools to strengthen the way we speak to others about who we are; allowing us to more accurately describe and promote our abilities and to step up our game.

Claiming expertise is useful for developing a great resumé and pitching for a next job. It is also useful in identifying personal strengths. Understanding these traits provides clarity for when to say "yes" and when to say "no" to new opportunities. Healthcare workers are often dealt *extra cards*. Knowing when to use or discard them makes a difference in how to play the game.

Reflecting on your personal *deck of success*, list all the roles you've had for five or more years—the roles in which you can claim to be an expert! Spend time creating your own one line commercial for what you do both personally and professionally. Practice saying it until it magically rolls off your tongue. Always remember your authenticity, creativity, and expertise make up your personal calling card and are the key to strength and power. Your ACE becomes an advantage and the center of your unique contribution; your *Ace in the hole.*

A POKER FACE HAS ITS PLACE

Designing Empathy

He looks like something that fell out of a deck of cards.

Bobby Human

Some people are simply not good at poker. Their faces give them away every time. That can be especially problematic for healthcare professionals.

Seeing, smelling, and hearing disgusting things; we aren't supposed to register shock or abhorrence. So, to be effective, we must put on a poker face. Patients can be brutalized by the fact that their bodies are betraying them and producing strange smells and sounds. If we don't show our disgust, we can make such trials easier to bear.

The ability for our faces and demeanors to reflect kindness and concern is essential for providing quality care. It's not simple and requires a great deal of practice. Sometimes our faces seem to have minds of their own, our eyes may betray us simply by narrowing a smidge, and the set of our mouth or jaw becomes as easily understood as a shout. It only takes an instant for a flicker of disinterest, contempt, or disgust to flitter across our faces.

A Traumatic Bluff

Understandably, healthcare professionals witness extraordinary things. Yet, our faces must remain neutral when confronted with wretched odors, bloody messes, and horrific tragedy. Patients and their families deserve our respect and that's reflected by our expressions and body language.

The last chapter discussed authenticity, and perhaps a poker face may seem a bit inauthentic. Yet, while we may register revulsion internally, this is not the time to let it appear on our faces. Being respectful necessitates putting on the poker face of kindness and concern. The higher value of serving humanity keeps us authentic.

The human experience of disease, illness, and tragedy require that we recognize the travails of the journey. In his book, *Radical Loving Care*, Erie Chapman suggests healthcare professionals recognize the patient gown as a cloak of respect that represents a "season of suffering." Considering the indignities of donning a hospital gown makes it easy to realize that someone is allowing healthcare providers to serve them in a unique and intimate way.

Hospital gowns are about as unattractive as any garment imaginable. One size fits all, and of course they don't. With only snaps to hold the front sides together, the back sides remain open and breezy. A cartoon depicts a guy wearing a patient gown glimpsing an image of his derriere as he passes a mirror. He states: "Now I know why they call this place, 'ICU!'"

Patients place deep trust in our care. As a patient donning the blue and white gown, and laying in a sterile white bed, made me realize I was simply another pale nameless person with all the personality of yesterday's cold oatmeal. Seeing through the eyes of a patient helped me become much more compassionate. And, that helped me start asking my patients what they are famous for. It provides a great way to learn more about their lives.

Viewing the hospital from a horizontal position is vastly different from working in the comfort of the vertical world. Spending endless hours in hospital beds and on gurneys encourages a patient's mind to drift to strange places and to ask odd questions. "Did someone die in this bed last night?" "Did something bad happen in this room?" "Oh horrors, will my body do something gross?" Caring about the suffering and humiliation of the patient, while seeing them as a human being in need, makes it much easier to remove our personal sensitivities and replace them with sincere concern. Maintaining a poker face helps.

Tell-Tale Emotions

During their sojourn in healthcare, patients and families are frequently given "bad news." Besides maintaining composure and a kind expression, finding a private place for the patient and family to digest their news is essential. Creating informative symbols to place on doorways to alert staff is helpful. Some hospitals use doves or butterflies to let staff know that a baby was born asleep. VA hospitals place a bald eagle portrait with a single tear drop on the door of the veteran who is dying. This not only alerts all staff to be sensitive, but also provides families with extra care and ensures appropriate conversations.

In serious situations, being informed can be essential to preventing emotional blunders. When lacking key information, the best thing a healthcare professional can do is simply listen.

After an early morning training session with labor and delivery nurses, Trudy stepped into the elevator with a middle-aged gentleman. He appeared totally exhausted, as if he'd been assisting his laboring wife all night. Trudy nearly asked, "so, is it a little girl or a little boy?" Yet, something told her that staying silent would be more appropriate. As the elevator door opened into the lobby, the man turned toward Trudy and said, "I'm trying to figure out how to say goodbye to my 21-year-old daughter who is not expected to live through the day." The next several minutes were spent in sincere and reflective listening to his heartbreaking story. As he left, he asked: "May I hug you? God put you on this elevator."

Healthcare workers have all witnessed inappropriate conversations and laughter at the front desk even while a physician is in an adjacent room delivering the "worst" news. That's not the time or place for even remotely insensitive behaviors. While on duty, we need to reflect appropriate concern. Later, after work or in the breakroom, we can find places where it's more appropriate to share our lives and celebrations with colleagues.

A poker face can also be beneficial when healthcare professionals have a disagreement with a new hire, colleague, or practitioner, especially when a patient or family member is within hearing range. Respectfully asking our colleague to step out of the room to an "off-stage" area to work through a disagreement is far better than appearing rude or getting upset in the presence of a patient.

One middle-aged, new grad shared a time when her supervisor sighed loudly, rolled her eyes in disgust, and snidely inquired: "What school of nursing did you say you graduated from?" The employee said she felt both attacked and betrayed. This supervisor could certainly have benefited by practicing her poker face, being nice, and practicing open feedback communication. It's always good to remember that, "more flies are caught by honey than vinegar." We experience more success by using simple common courtesy.

To develop great communication and trustworthy teamwork requires healthcare professionals to find out what the student, new hire, or colleague was thinking, feeling, and seeing in a situation. Each of us sees life and events from a unique perspective.

Attempting to understand the other person first, listening completely, and then openly thanking the person for sharing their perspective, allows professionals to express their thoughts and have their voices heard. Someone who listens well earns the right to ask the other person if they are open to feedback. This method is nearly always successful. A respectful poker face whenever a person may be struggling with difficult emotions opens up communication.

Saving Face

After my teenage son was hired as an emergency department tech in a large medical center, he arrived home following a shift with eyes wide. "Mom," he blurted. "You'd never imagine what happened last night. A most disgusting man came in."

While I put on a pot of coffee, my son continued his story. "He was physically filthy and his mood was filthy. Even his words were filthy. I was so disgusted, especially with the way he treated the nurse!"

I nodded, "I know. Some people have lived through things we know nothing about."

My son continued, "You'll never guess what happened. His nurse quietly went and got two basins of water and started bathing him. I couldn't believe it. I asked why she did that, because we don't bathe patients in emergency." He took a sip of coffee and continued "She simply answered: 'I have to take care of him for 12 hours, and I'd rather take care of a clean patient than a dirty one.'"

This wonderful nurse easily could have delegated the task of bathing her patient to my son. Instead, she showed him a priceless example.

As a homecare nurse, I've had plenty of practice slapping on a poker face. I still remember approaching a patient's house one hot and muggy afternoon in July. The plants and vines intertwined making it feel like I was entering a cave. While scanning the porch for spiders, I knocked tentatively.

A middle-aged lady, the Miz, opened the door, greeted me, and had me enter a small stoop. In the center of the room, a beautiful elderly lady with silver hair swept up elegantly and held in place by a big gold bow sat in a wheelchair. By the referral I recognized my patient. I quickly noted that her oxygen was being delivered appropriately, and she seemed alert and oriented. The next sensation was an overpowering stench of cat urine.

Looking around the room, I noted an oilcloth on the floor with multiple bowls of cat food, chairs piled high with papers and magazines, a table loaded with dirty dishes, and a flocked Christmas tree with red bows and twinkling white lights. Miz appeared to preside from an overstuffed white chair next to it.

A later visit found the Miz ranting and raving that someone was trying to kill "her" as she jabbed a finger toward her mother. I queried further as to "who" would want to kill this lovely lady and was told emphatically that it was either "Burt Reynolds or her son!" As this visit proceeded, my patient's hand gestured for me to move near. Then, she whispered: "Miz is schizophrenic!"

On my last visit, the Miz inquired as to where I usually purchased my Christmas tree. Evidently, she was having great difficulty finding a "flocked" tree. She pointed to her sad, twinkling tree and said she hadn't found a good one since Nurseryland had closed, three years prior.

Yikes! This wasn't an old artificial tree. It was a totally dead "real" one!

My patient was on oxygen and the fire threat was high. Fearing for her safety, I called the local fire department. Using my best HIPPA language I told them they may have a fire hazard on Maple Street. I shared the story of the dried-up Christmas tree and the patient on oxygen. Suddenly the fire captain exclaimed, "Oh, you mean the house with too many cats!"

Caring for my lovely elderly patient and the Miz gave me many opportunities to act with kindness and genuine concern. A lesson for success is knowing when a *poker face has its place*. If we have a heart of service towards those we are privileged to care for, we will master our faces and reflect appropriate respect whether we're facing challenging sights, emotions, or concerns.

SHUFFLE THE DECK

Accepting Change and Discovering Opportunities

Whether you're shuffling a deck of cards or holding your breath, magic is pretty simple: It comes down to training, practice, and experimentation, followed up by ridiculous pursuit and relentless perseverance.

David Blaine

To play a good and fair game, the cards must be well-shuffled. Without that, card games become predictable and boring. Observing people shuffle a deck is fascinating. Some do it with fanfare. Others end up with 52 card pickup. Sometimes an electronic device is used to accomplish the feat.

Healthcare has similar options. Some team members are skilled at shuffling and prioritizing a multifaceted workload. Others have a real challenge identifying the priority balance and seem unable to shift away from a preset task list.

Many electronic tools and applications are available to support the practitioners, who find shifting priorities difficult. Often these electronic applications, though well-intentioned, don't enhance a level of competence and flexibility. Healthcare professionals, who have achieved great skill shuffling responsibilities, are challenged to share their techniques with colleagues who may be struggling.

Shuffling Workloads

To be effective, healthcare team members must become skilled at shifting task assignments whenever necessary. Patient acuity levels continually change and admissions, discharges, and workflow patterns ebb and flow throughout a shift. In clinics, service departments, and outpatient facilities—patient flow can be challenging to balance.

Physicians and other practitioners, with joint responsibilities in both hospitals and clinics, find shuffling the needs of everyone, daunting. The sickest must be prioritized, and that can delay meeting the needs of those with appointments. How a healthcare team communicates with its guests in these situations is critical to providing good customer service and patient-friendly perceptions. Emergency departments, now accessed as a portal to primary care, find themselves with many new patients while "holding" other patients awaiting admission. This becomes an extreme shuffling game.

Those who have mastered skills in this type of flexibility need to find ways to pass them on to those new to healthcare or who lack expertise in this area. Shuffling a schedule requires practice and constant fine-tuning. Acknowledging the challenges does not make someone unworthy of a healthcare career, nor does it demonstrate a lack of education. Rather it is a skill that needs to be mastered. Asking for feedback and continually practicing new approaches can help someone master this skill.

Shuffling Positions

Learning to mix things up for your own personal satisfaction is also a valuable skill. It's important to acknowledge when stress within a job and/or your personal life requires attention. You are the best one to recognize when this is happening. Learning your boundaries, energy levels, and capabilities is critical to preventing "burn out!"

Identifying personal goals and creating plans to move toward accomplishment of those goals is important. Some colleagues wait for work or something else in their lives to change, rather than seeking ways to improve their position or finding work that better suits them. Yet, they need to shuffle their own decks because employers won't do it for them. Don't wait for someone to offer a change—go after what you want.

Once, at a staff recognition banquet, I ran into a colleague I'd worked with early in my career. During our conversation, I asked where she was currently working. Shockingly, she was on the very same unit where we had worked twenty-five years previously.

Perhaps longevity in one area speaks well of employee satisfaction; but perhaps, it speaks of complacency. It is not our employer's responsibility to move us forward in our career. In fact, our employers encourage us to stay in the same position. They do not want us to leave our role as it's costly to replace us; therefore, they may not honor our goals for growth.

Shuffling your own deck ensures that you work in the areas of your strengths and giftedness. Lesson 5, "Claim Your ACE" encourages you to identify and learn your strengths. It is counterproductive to work in your weaknesses. Working in your areas of expertise and creativity makes work enjoyable and prevents burn-out.

Gallup's *StrengthsFinder 2.0* by Tom Rath recognizes 34 leadership strengths. Every person has five dominant strengths from which to draw his greatest energy and talent. Knowing your strengths and gifts helps you know when to say "yes" and when to say "no."

Some leaders challenge their teams to identify and improve their weaknesses. Gallup contends a weakness is not something you cannot do; nor is it something you cannot do well. However; a weakness is something that in the doing, exhausts you and drains you dry. Ideally, you should be spending 80 percent of your day working in your strength. When working in an area of strength, the day flows. Often the job a healthcare professional is initially hired for morphs into something entirely different. Looking at the *hand you were dealt* and assessing if it has changed greatly is highly advisable. When your position no longer supports your strengths, it may be time to *shuffle* your *deck* and look for work that aligns with your goals and talents.

Organizational Shuffles

Sometimes our deck of cards gets shuffled for us. An administration changes, the hospital or clinic is sold, the goals and values of an organization are redefined and it seems that we are suddenly playing a new game. Healthcare regulations change and simultaneously a workplace strategy may be altered.

Organizations have every right to change course. Employees also have the right to decide on a new direction. After a new hand is dealt, it's important to assess what is going well and what causes concern.

In his book, *Good to Great*, Jim Collins draws a parallel of organizational direction to that of a bus. If a bus changes direction, an employee has several options. The first recommendation is to simply sit down and look around. That way the employee can get a feel for the new route—to understand the "why" behind the change in the direction and consider the following:

- What changed?

- Does this new direction align with my values?

- Do these changes impact me personally?

- Can I continue to support the direction of this organization?

- How does this new direction support or detract from the care I provide to my patients?

- Are these changes creating more or less safety for patients and myself?

Asking a great question is more important than finding a quick answer. Sometimes it takes more than one answer to discover the best option. The second or third answer may offer a more inspired way of thinking. Often it is well past the fourth idea, that solutions start to appear.

After riding the bus in the new direction for awhile, it may be time to see if a different seat offers a better vantage point. Crisis and change within an organization can present the prime circumstances to strategically move into a new area. Chaos can bring unprecedented opportunity. Once everything settles down, organizations usually revert to a slow and methodical routine.

If the situation has been adequately assessed, the best solution may be to simply run toward the nearest escape route to get off the bus. An employee always has the power to make choices. He is not at the mercy of the organization where he works. When it comes to a significant change, he can either accept it, fix it, forget it, or leave it!

Although surviving an organizational *shuffle* may not feel good in the moment, many employees are happier afterwards. And in the midst of the *shuffle*, they can do something that adds value to their roles and their organization. Wise healthcare professionals resist the temptation to whine, point fingers, or gossip. And if they choose to leave the organization, do so with grace and dignity. Being disrespectful, even if someone doesn't deserve your respect, rarely pays off. Taking the high road *pays off in spades*!

Mixing It Up Myself

One of the shuffles I experienced happened while I was working as an educator in a large home-health organization. I enjoyed my work immensely and knew I was contributing to the success of the organization. Then, a subtle shift created a disturbing undercurrent. It seemed like some of the administrators in the parent organization were not fully valuing the work being accomplished by the department.

At year end, it was my practice to take stock of my results and focus on writing goals for the upcoming year. I sat before my computer ready to establish educational goals for the department. Suddenly I drew a blank. I stared at the computer for the better part of two days—nothing—nada. I couldn't write a single goal.

Randomly my fingers typed, "your job is to find a new job!" Voila! Within five minutes I had listed ten things I wanted and needed in a new job. With the new list in hand, I phoned a friend and asked if she knew of a job that matched my list. In less than a week, I landed my dream job as a staff development education specialist.

I'm not naive enough to believe we always get what we want or deserve. Living through a monumental organizational shuffle provided quite a different experience. This one was a "workplace divorce!" I had been recruited to bring education, leadership, and orientation expertise to a hospital that had already endured a great deal of leadership turmoil. Our team had made two years of steady progress until suddenly the gossip grapevine began to vibrate.

Within the space of eight weeks, all the C-Suite leadership positions had been vacated through a series of resignations. The parent organization quickly filled those positions with temporary, contract leadership. Staff vulnerability was high, trust was broken, and anxiety palpably rippled through the halls.

As the weeks progressed, meetings were canceled. The new leadership team did not talk to mid-level managers. Rumors of layoffs abounded. My fellow leaders and my personal team all felt threatened. Fear replaced creativity and productivity.

I told my husband that I feared I may be fired. He was shocked. He reminded me of my strong reputation with the parent organization and my large sphere of influence. I replied, "living on one's 'laurels' doesn't appear to be helpful." Friday afternoon layoffs in middle management had become the norm. One Monday night, it was my turn to be part of the reduction in force ("RIF," a fancy acronym for being laid off).

Through that experience I learned—no matter how prepared a person thinks she is to be let go, she is not. Earlier on that fateful day, my team had asked if they should fear for their jobs. I had suggested that I should be the one laid off as my services were not being well-utilized. Yet when it happened, I was stunned.

To receive severance, I was not allowed to say goodbye to my team. I was told to pack my office, then was walked to my car. I felt like a criminal. Someone in management reminded me of my great performance record and reassured me that he was very sorry. It didn't help. Neither did the reassurance of my eligibility for immediate rehire in another role. Colleagues who also experienced pink slips, RIFs, and unfair layoffs validated my feelings.

Over the weeks, I came to view this shuffle much like a divorce. In a familial divorce, there are times when a mutual decision is reached and both parties agree to the outcome. At other times divorce is unilateral. One person decides to break the relationship blindsiding the other person. Or one person secretively decides to break the relationship, yet their spouse has seen indicators or suspects that things are amiss.

All three of these situations also occur in the workplace, and many of the same feelings arise—loss, anger, distrust, discouragement, low self-esteem, depression, and self-doubt. In a workplace divorce; a person loses friends, attachments, career prestige, and much of what brought meaning to life.

This final shuffle style can also provide opportunities to do things differently. Perhaps it's time to stop working for a corporation. For several years, I had dreamed and planned a career move that would permit me to speak, teach, consult, and write. I had created a mission statement and key focus areas. I was determined to inspire women (the primary purveyors and purchasers of healthcare), to unleash passion, purpose, and power.

Though I wanted to provide coaching for nurse leaders, especially those in frontline and middle management, I found myself hesitant to step out on my own. Fear of the unknown held me back. Staying stuck in a job that pays well, provides great benefits, and has a perception of security can create a great deal of complacency.

As I've interviewed people, who have moved through similar conundrums, I've found that we interpret job loss based on our values and beliefs. Some people identify unexpected opportunities to care for children or elderly parents. Early retirement and travel offer a positive outlook for some. Others lose their identity, which was based in the profession that grounded them. I've also talked to those who experienced a profound loss of self-esteem and financial security. It may take them many resumes and interviews to land their next job. They tell of being torn away from family and community by having to move across the country for new career opportunities.

As for me, I needed to grapple with the values and mission of the organization to which I had devoted most of my career. I struggled with feelings of betrayal, profound loss, and professional irrelevance. I've learned that while individuals can usually be counted on to reflect their own core values, corporations are businesses not people. While a business may have mission, vision, and values statements; they have no feeling.

When a carefully constructed *house of cards* topples, it's important to embrace the uncertainty and look for opportunities, some of which may be difficult to recognize. Author Brene Brown, inspires us to "choose courage over comfort." Quite often, mixing it up takes courage, yet embracing change or even creating it will bring great rewards.

Now, I am building my career on a different foundation. For a decade, I'd been dreaming and planning the construction of a "remodeled" career. Yet I lacked the guts to step out on my own. Stepping away from my corporate identity has taken bravery, creativity, and perseverance. On occasion, the magnet still tugs toward the comfort of my nursing position supported by the hospital who employed me.

I have had to learn to trust my ACE of talents, my expertise, and the good will of my circles of influence. Landing smack dab in the middle of a career overhaul has taught me a lot about myself. I've learned remodels:

- take way longer than anticipated

- cost way more than budgeted

- get far messier than our wildest imagination

Through it all, my personal mantra has been the word: "Plenty!" I've realized I have plenty of family, friends, talents, abilities, and resources. And, I survived! I've built a thriving speaking, coaching, and consulting career. My past experiences blended with my personal strengths helped me forge a new pathway into my mission and purpose.

CLOSE TO THE VEST OR FACE UP

Effective Communication

I'm not a poker player. I'm not a bluff. My way is to look someone in the eye and tell them the way I'm intending to go. My cards are always on the table.

Tori Amos

Cards. Knowing when to hold and when to fold makes all the difference between winning and losing. When poker stakes get high, a cardsharp puts on a poker face and holds his cards carefully—away from prying eyes. That's called playing *close to the vest*. A cardsharp never lets anyone see his cards nor will he give his position away with body language. He may be holding a winning hand and hope others believe that they are losing or vice versa. That's called *bluffing*.

But when we teach people to play a new game of cards, we might play *face up*. Teaching and learning become more important than winning. Cards are dealt to everyone and, in turn, the players lay their cards face up so that each individual hand can be seen. Then, it's easy to demonstrate how to play the most favorable cards without worrying about how that impacts the next player. On around the table it goes, so the new player can understand the game's strategy.

Keeping Information "Close to the Vest"

In healthcare, there's many reasons to keep a strategy concealed. Success for staff members, leaders, patient advocates, or any team player comes by understanding when and how to communicate. Healthcare professionals often receive information that is not theirs to share.

At other times, providing information can mean life or death. Learning when and how to communicate clearly may determine whether a patient lives or dies.

Playing close to the vest is an appropriate strategy for frontline or mid-level leaders, who are privy to information not to be shared with staff. Understanding the rationale behind appropriate framing and timing of a message is an essential component of good leadership.

Too often, administrators fail to recognize the great responsibility they have in communicating important messages to the organization. Instead of creating a strategy, clarity of messaging, and a precise timeline, they allow each leader to share what "feels right!" Such a failure of planning and strategizing leads to the grapevine effect. Allowing people to collect partial knowledge and apply their own spin to the story usually creates enormous distortions. On the other hand, careful crafting of a message focused on the direct effects to the employee is the administration's responsibility, not frontline or mid-level leadership.

By way of example, one hospital administration made the decision to enhance the patient experience by using an evidence-based practice. Everyone at the table agreed to place employees in a preselected color of scrub apparel. The reasoning was simple—avoiding confusion for the patients and their families. They could easily distinguish, by the color of the uniform, who or what service was providing their care.

Unfortunately, the administration made this decision by committee. And, before making the decision, they spoke only to other leaders, not the employees, who would be most impacted. Though the leadership clearly saw the advantages, they failed to recognize the effects of this decision on employees. Because they were the ones being told what to wear, they cared and reacted.

The grapevine began buzzing with misinformation. Anger and resentment percolated. As part of the "change management roll-out team," I was asked to deliver the message in large group meetings. And, that's when the employees' anger and resentment boiled over.

The initial mandate required every employee to purchase their own "color" and employees expressed their displeasure: "They tried this a few years ago, and it failed." "We will ensure it fails again." "I will lay low and not buy my uniform until it blows over."

As the dissension mounted, the administration retrenched and purchased the scrubs. Upon reflection, if the message had been managed more effectively, it could have been framed for success. First, the administrators needed to recognize what was at stake in demanding a clothing choice and color for the employees. Second, they could have framed the action by clearly articulating the concerns for patient safety and satisfaction. Third, by purchasing and embroidering the scrubs with the company logo, administrators would have created a valuable win for teamwork. Fourth, to ensure success as well as enhance employee recognition, the administration could have also embroidered the employee's name on the scrub shirt just below the logo. Employees then would have seen this effort as a gift and might have embraced the concept whole-heartedly.

There are many great reasons to hold information close until a more appropriate time. Employees do not need to know the pros and cons of many decisions. However, it is imperative that key decisions are communicated quickly and clearly. Messages should be framed for success from the employee's point of view, so they don't come across as the results of an administrative whim.

And, when a communicated decision needs to be changed or reversed, that message must clearly state the rationale. Too often messages are blasted out to "all employee groups" via email, only to be followed by several additional e-mails to clarify. This can be confusing and counterproductive. If administrators and committee chairs take a few additional minutes to carefully craft the content of their messages, while considering their impact, timing, and potential for push-back—many problems could be alleviated.

There are also times when a healthcare professional is required to withhold bad news from a patient, and that can be especially tough.

During my senior year of nursing school, I was assigned a surgical patient who I would be caring for throughout her entire surgical stay—from pre-op to scrubbing in on the surgical procedure, then on to the post-surgical unit. Mrs. Collins was a 57-year-old suffering upper-right-quadrant belly pain. She was scheduled for a cholecystectomy, gallbladder surgery. At the time, a gallbladder surgery was rigorous and required a minimum of four-to-five days in the hospital with all the attendant drains and tubes.

Upon entering her room, I encountered a vivacious lady dressed in a beautiful robe with coiffed hair and manicured nails. We reviewed the pre-operative nursing assessment, and I assured her I'd be with her the entire time she was in surgery.

During the procedure, the physician announced that the patient not only had a compromised gall bladder, but worse, a "hobnail" liver indicative of advanced cirrhosis and cancer. He said he could do nothing surgically to save this patient. Then he looked right at me, and said: "Little nurse, I do not want you to tell this patient anything about what you have seen and learned today. I will discuss the outcome at her first office visit because I want her to have time to heal before she receives the bad news."

I struggled with this request as my patient kept asking, "did you see my gallstones?" I felt the physician's request was unreasonable. It challenged my authenticity and ability to be truthful. I was being asked to withhold critical information, and it didn't feel right. In this case, however, I needed to submit my feelings to the surgeon's judgment and play it close to the vest.

A few months later, assignments were posted on the medical floor. My stomach lurched, and my emotions reeled as I saw Mrs. Collins' name on my patient list. How could I go into her room? Surely, she'd be angry with me! She had every right to hate me, as I had withheld the truth from her. How dare my instructor assign her case to me?

After several long moments, I realized I could not put off the inevitable and quietly crept into her room. What a change a few weeks had made! She was very ill, emaciated, and comatose. Her family surrounded her and kept urging her to "hang on" a few more hours until her son could arrive.

I still remember feeling an odd mixture of relief and guilt, all swirled together. I was able to meet the needs of the family without meeting the accusing eyes of my patient. Thinking back on this event, I still struggle with the dilemma of whether it's best to keep difficult news *close to the vest* or *face up* when it comes to patients and their families. All health-care providers must grapple with this dilemma.

Conveying Information "Face Up"

Some staff members seem to have no verbal filters and "blab" everything without considering the impact to those within hearing distance. This is the negative side of laying your cards on the table. It's a phenomenon that can easily be observed at front desks in hospitals, in clinics, and other medical offices. Overheard by the wrong person, conversations emanating from behind desks have the potential to be devastating.

Hallway gossip is also prevalent in many healthcare settings. While the comradery of staff is usually beneficial, healthcare professionals must be vigilant that while "on stage," the conversation should be appropriate. Patients and their family members do not want to know what happened in Las Vegas last week. Additionally, guests can easily interpret an overheard conversation to be about them, whether that's true or not. And, when staff speak to each other in a foreign language, everyone around, including other staff members, may believe the conversation is about them.

Having an off-stage area, such as a breakroom, provides a place where staff can have personal conversations. A private place is also extremely valuable when a staff member needs to step away from a situation to shake off frustration, anger, or other negative emotions. The ability to move from situation to situation rapidly, without carrying over feelings, is a skill and competence each healthcare professional must hone.

On the positive side, conveying information with the cards *face up* is often the best approach when communicating within a team. They need to know what to expect from their leaders and colleagues. By being honest when experiencing a difficult day, others can step up and cross monitor a situation. It is essential that teams know their leaders are not *bluffing* and can be depended upon for straightforward communication.

Trust, as described in Lesson 3: "Every Card is Valuable", is essential to good teamwork. A team leader builds trust by being open and honest while providing clear communication. Consistent actions convey congruence with a spoken message, and that *stacks the deck* in a team's favor.

> Using "I" statements is an excellent training tool
> for delivering positive messages:
>
> I feel [e.g., upset] _____
>
> When [e.g., I think a patient isn't being taken care of] _____
>
> Because [e.g., it scares me that infection might set in] _____
>
> I need/ I want you to [e.g., check that dressing every hour] ___
>
> This non-threatening communication style opens the way for en-hanced understanding and clarity.

Many healthcare organizations have adopted the TeamSTEPPS method of communication. This methodology provides many essentials to reduce miscommunication and error. TeamSTEPPS communication is a Department of Defense strategy that is being utilized by healthcare to improve patient safety. Many organizations are utilizing its components to enhance communication across multi-team systems. Terms that may be familiar include SBAR, call out, hand off, situation monitoring and two-challenge rule. For more information, follow www.ahrq.gov/teamstepps.

As healthcare providers embrace this universal language, there's an increase in effective communication. Mastery of these techniques is a life-long struggle that must be diligently assessed and constantly worked on.

Physicians, advanced practice nurses, physician assistants, and others in the healing profession also have the challenge of communicating difficult messages to families and patients. On every healthcare team, someone struggles with the best way to share the "bad news," just as that physician (and I) did with Mrs. Collins. And, sometimes families and/or patients request that pieces of "bad news," not be shared. This creates a very delicate dance of how to hold the cards in our hands.

At times we lay all the cards on the table. As when teaching a card game, face up is imperative for learning and collaboration. In fact, it is probably the best way for healthcare teams to work together effectively. Clear communication is essential. Allowing others to guess what we are thinking, needing, or wanting is a sure-fire way to be misunderstood.

Open communication lets patients and their families know what to expect and their role in self-care. It also permits them to make their wishes known. Much of healthcare is about influencing patients to make changes in their own health. Healthcare providers simply cannot be responsible for the long-term health of another person. We can only do our best in the current situation.

It is up to the patient and their family to make choices and take responsibility for themselves. They can't be forced to change. So, education is essential. Helping an individual understand the consequences of his choices is vital. It then becomes his responsibility.

Clinicians often speak about how "we" will manage someone's diabetes, for example. If the patient is in the hospital and their food is measured and medications administered by the nurse, perhaps healthcare professionals can make the claim that "we" manage her diabetes. However, once the patient goes home, only she can manage her diabetes. All healthcare practitioners can do is share information so the person can make her own informed choices.

A great example of this happened when my elderly mother suffered a severe bout of weakness leaving her suddenly unable to ambulate or care for herself. When I took her to our local urgent care, we were met by a most amazing staff of caring and compassionate nurses and physicians. The entire team showed great respect to an elderly woman.

Unfortunately, this is often not the case. Aging creates a barrier of invisibility and subsequently devalues a suffering human being. In our situation, the urgent care physician spoke English as a second language; however, he paced his speech and enunciation with such care that my German mother clearly understood him.

The lab results showed respiratory and kidney failure—not a good omen. An internal medicine physician was called. Again, the professionalism, crisp lab coat, and attentive manner of this physician exceeded all expectations. After greeting my mother and asking a few pertinent questions, he asked if she had advance directives. I replied that indeed she did and at the generous age of 93, my mother would want kind, respectful, and dignified comfort care.

He explained that he could support the kidney failure by providing my mother with significant fluids; however, the action would most definitely compromise the respiratory failure which could be managed with intubation. My response was clear, "No we wouldn't put her through that kind of suffering."

He followed, "I can manage your mother's respiratory failure by giving diuretics, but that will compromise the kidneys—however, we can manage that by dialysis." He then looked tenderly at my mother and patted her gently on the shoulder. Shaking his head, he offered, "I suspect a woman of this age would not tolerate dialysis well."

In an attempt to balance the fluid load, Mother was admitted for two days. The physician phoned every morning to talk over the plan of care. When it became apparent that treatment goals were not achievable, we opted to take Mother home and put her on hospice. The physician urged for a late-evening discharge, which seemed odd to the family. Wouldn't tomorrow morning be easier?

The physician's greatest concern for discharge was that he was going off duty at midnight and didn't want to turn her care over to a new team. He knew the oncoming team would not have had the privilege and understanding afforded through our many conversations. He feared they might repeat unnecessary testing and care cycles.

The communication, goals, and understanding the physician and family had attained were remarkable. As he left the room for a final time, he shook our hands and said, "I wish I could have this kind of conversation and respectful decision making with all my patients and their families." It was clear, decisions had been made with all the information on the table. That made a profound difference in the care we received.

When considering the best way to play a hand, either *close to the vest* or *face up*—taking the time necessary to reflect on the desired results, the impact on the team and/or the patient, and the value added to those involved is essential. Finding that perfect "think spot," for journaling or taking courses in communication will create mastery in decision-making skills. Spending personal reflective time—whether at the beginning or the end of the day—to evaluate when, where, and how to communicate will turn that communication into a priceless gift.

LESSON 9

EVERY DAY, LIFE DEALS A NEW HAND

Developing Resilience

Each player must accept the cards life deals him or her; but once they are in the hand, he or she alone must decide how to play the cards in order to win the game.

Voltaire

The good news is that healthcare professionals have choices. We have the ability to do something different today than the way we did it yesterday. The past is past. Today is here and tomorrow is a promissory note. Conversations today create our tomorrows.

Once, especially as young adults, we asked so many questions about the "what ifs!" Many of these questions are deeply rooted in the larger question of how will making a particular decision impact ourselves, our families, our careers, and our friendships. We wonder how our future will unfold if we make choice "A" over choice "B."

When we are choosing our career:

- "What if I decide to become a nurse instead of a physician?"

- "What if I select therapy over becoming an engineer?"

- "What if I select a residency on the east coast vs. the Midwest?"

With more experience, the questions change:

- "Who might be affected if I decide I don't want to do this?"

- "How will a new job affect my financial future?"

- "What can I do to be a better practitioner?"

- "Should I return for an advanced degree or certification?"

Later in life, questions change once again.

- "Would it be better if I retire at 62 or 75?"

- How can I leave a legacy within my career field?"

- Can I use my experience, gifts, and talents to create a new future for myself?

No one has a crystal ball that can predict the future. An individual's choices (along with the *luck of the draw*) create their future. Most of what we worry about, never even comes to pass. That's why the "what ifs" must not stop a person from moving forward and accepting the results that she wants to achieve. The bottom line is—all decisions create a direction; however, the roadmap is not yet written. We make our best decision and move forward.

It was in the midst of thinking about these things, that I came to realize how life mimics a good game of cards. And, the concept became clear that every single day life deals each of us a fresh hand of new cards.

Each day as physicians, nurses, or therapists; we pick up our hands and *read 'em or weep.* Though we hope for a winner, we realize it could be a mess. Then there's the hope that lady luck will help us. Yet sometimes, despite our hopes and dreams, we might be dealt a lousy hand. Then we may want to just fold and walk away.

All life asks for is that we play the hand we are given to the best of our ability. No more or less is required. Tomorrow everyone is dealt another hand.

A Full House

There's no dilemma with a great hand. We simply enjoy it and recognize the gift that it is. The minute we receive: a great promotion, the opportunity to assist the chief surgeon with a highly technical surgery, a great residency—we can appreciate the possibilities and express our gratitude.

When I was in my mid-twenties and nearing the end of graduate school. I was struggling with decisions on how to finance my out-of-country internship, cover my rent, and take an unpaid leave from my job as an emergency department charge nurse. About midnight the phone rang and the caller asked if I would consider leaving my emergency room position to become the training coordinator of the Paramedic Program for the School of Medicine. "Oh yes," he added, "can you let us know by tomorrow morning?" Questions poured out of me:

- "You mean like Gage and DeSoto on Rescue 911?"........"Yes."

- "Is there a curriculum?"....... ....No."

- "Who else has done this?" ...."Dr. Stewart in LA County."

- "Has it been done in the Inland Empire?" ...."No."

- "Have students have been selected?"...... "Yes, 26 fire fighters are ready."

- "Do I have a boss?"........"Yes and no—he won't be around for six weeks."

- "What about my graduate internship?".........."We will find a solution!"

- "I've never taught. How do you know I can do this?" ...."All we need is your enthusiasm!" (Later, I learned that was a fable!)

Playing that winning hand well, I said yes to an amazing journey. It was not; however, without challenges. My office was an apple box in the trunk of my car. The first session, I was never more than one day ahead of my students in planning and executing the curriculum.

The morning I started the second cohort, I couldn't seem to stop crying and shaking. I realized how emotionally challenging the first session had been. Then, I looked at some additional cards I'd been dealt. Another instructor had been added to my team to support the next cohort of first responders.

During the time that I coordinated the Paramedic Program, many people came alongside to ensure my success. Nurse educators from the School of Nursing helped me select textbooks and create curriculum. Dr. Stewart, father of Paramedicine, Los Angeles County, University of Southern California (LAC-USC), handed me a six-inch thick mimeographed binder of his materials stating: "What's mine is yours."

Firefighter students shared their lecture notes and gave me plenty of feedback on what was right and what was seriously wrong with my tests and curriculum. Physician leaders gave me access to their senior residents who participated as guest lecturers. Nurse leaders allowed my students full access to clinical learning. Fire chiefs across San Bernardino and Los Angeles Counties provided internships within their facilities

Looking back on this experience, I'm amazed at the opportunity and trust that was placed in me. I often say it was "trial by fire!" Standing in front of all those firefighter students toughened me up in a hurry.

A Pair of Nines

Learning from the daily hand helps us repeat success. Some days we can be so distracted we may miss the great hand we've been dealt. Unfortunately, once it is played, no matter if you played well or poorly, it cannot be salvaged.

This lesson also reminds us to be in the moment. Living in the past or fretting over regrets keeps us from living the day we truly have. Worrying about tomorrow and something that is yet to exist robs us of the present, as well. When we give in to F.E.A.R. of the future, we are allowing ourselves to focus on "False Evidence Appearing Real!" Truth be told, less than 95 percent of what we fear and fret about ever becomes reality. Fear is a thief!

Most days our cards are simply mediocre. On those days we may be tempted to coast, to not pay attention. Yet by focusing and always putting forth our best efforts, we cultivate the winning opportunities that may appear in the future. And, occasionally a mediocre hand still wins the game. Seeing life within the framework of possibility is an art. Changing our perspective allows us to see a new horizon. Bad news isn't always all bad. With every challenge comes an equal or greater opportunity.

At dinner one night, my friend, Tom, a heavy equipment operator, was bemoaning the current economic environment and relating the struggles his company was having. Suddenly he cried out, "What we need is another Northridge earthquake!" Everyone erupted into shouts: "Are you crazy?"

"Not really," he replied, "Several years ago our company was nearly bankrupt and then the Northridge earthquake hit, and we had all kinds of work to repair the bridges that were damaged." While I'm certainly not suggesting that we hope for calamity, even within moments of loss and chaos, we can find opportunities by simply looking for them.

No Suits, No Runs, No Face Cards

Sometimes, though, no matter how hard we try, life gives us a really bad *hand*, or worse, maybe we miss or bungle a great opportunity. Is that a game changer? Most likely, yes. Even so, we can't worry about it. Always there's the hope that tomorrow brings.

Jim, a successful middle-aged businessman, shared what seemed like a disaster when it first happened, but took on great meaning over time. He was clearly not winning a ravaging battle against cancer. One night, as the oncology nurse was tucking her patients into bed, he reached out and grabbed her arm, asking: "Can I share with you the blessing cancer has been to me?"

Hearing such unusual words, she pulled up a chair and sat down. She listened as he described his frantically busy life. It was full of all the perks that success, wealth, and travel provide. Then he received a sobering diagnosis.

"In the past five years," Jim said, "everything has changed. I've had the opportunity to reconnect with my friends and tell them how much they've meant to me. I've spent time with my children listening to their dreams, watching them grow, and ensuring they have the tools and skills necessary to succeed without me. And, I've had the chance to fall in love with my wife, all over again!"

This story reminds us that every day we get to choose our perspective. Our feelings come upon us unbidden, however, the way we view them and the behavior we select creates our attitude. And, attitude has a great deal to do with the altitude we'll reach.

It's also true that old hands cannot be replayed. Once a hand has been dealt and played—it's game over. For those who have lived through turbulent healthcare administrations, been part of system-wide layoffs, or been unfairly dismissed—there is a temptation to dwell in the inequity of the event. Most often we experience feelings of anger, hurt, broken trust, and depression. We question what our loyalty meant. Yet, life continues with forward momentum. Though memories can be indulged for a brief moment, those circumstances no longer exist; and it's best to treasure the good, learn from the not-so-good, and move on.

Stepping into your new future is a sign that healing is occurring. Embracing new opportunities and new colleagues can bring unexpected restoration. To feel valued and appreciated allows us to embrace the future.

REMEMBER THE SUITS

Treating People Well and Respecting Their Journey

The simplest way to say it is that I think we're all dealt these cards in life, but the cards in and of themselves don't read one way or the other. It's up to you to home [sic] in and cultivate whatever you've got in your hand.

Pharrell Williams

Before starting this final lesson, a summary of the first nine lessons of the cards will help us keep them in mind:

1. ***Rules change but the cards don't.*** While healthcare is experiencing tremendous amounts of change and our work-world is in constant disruption, our patients continue to trust and depend on our expertise and advocacy.

2. ***While you can't cure everyone, you can heal many.*** Those who are suffering from disease and trauma seek the care of healthcare professionals. We provide solutions and fixes when possible. Yet we must recognize our limitations in providing physical and emotional cures. Finding spaces for meaningful conversations, for seeking understanding, and offering solace amid suffering is healing.

3. *Every card is valuable.* Respecting the contributions, gifts, and talents of every individual on the healthcare team is vital. Our unique teams are composed of professional and nonprofessional members. And, together we are what the patient needs most.

4. *Integrity makes you a great player.* When we establish our integrity, we have a framework for decision making. Faced with a challenging situation, our internal compass will be set for correct action. Other team members will respect and trust us.

5. *Claiming your ACE gives you an advantage.* Leveraging our accountability, creativity, and expertise ensures that we are a valuable member of the team. We are able to speak to our strengths and talents and declare ourselves in service to our patients and colleagues.

6. *A poker face has its place.* Designing empathy into our practice is essential. Learning to cope with horrific trauma and serious disease ramifications while providing respectful, dignified care to our patients is a sacred trust.

7. *Shuffle the deck.* By accepting change, you can discover opportunities. Managing variable workloads, patient needs, and work flows takes skill acquisition. Finding the right career path may require the deck to be shuffled. When someone else shuffles the deck, we need to take a step back and consider the opportunities.

8. *When communicating, you can keep information close to the vest or face up.* Effective communication is an essential competence for healthcare professionals. There is a place for safeguarding information and a time for transparency. Mastering communication skills requires us to do more listening and less talking.

9. *Life deals you a new hand every day.* Resilience or grit is the ability to recover quickly from difficulty. We can learn to count our blessings and determine when to stand strong. Finding our inner strength happens when our heads connect with our hearts. And, by accepting that this day is all we have.

Now for the final lesson—drum roll please!

REMEMBER THE SUITS 119

Lesson # 10. Remember the Suits

The four suits in a deck of cards set an appropriate standard for how to treat people in respectful relationships. These basic principles add value to every encounter. When healthcare professionals apply them, the need for customer service training is diminished. And, remembering the points in this lesson is as simple as remembering the different suits in a deck of cards.

Like a Diamond

Healthcare professionals need to try to see every individual as being a diamond. Some diamonds sparkle and are highly polished. These are easy to spot. Yet others are still "in the rough."

Several sources bring forth diamonds, but most start forming deep in the earth or sea. Surrounded by volcanic debris called kimberlite, finding them requires a highly skilled eye.

Diamonds experience tremendous heat and pressure in order to crystalize the carbon. Then following a long extraction process, they are crushed and sorted by color, weight, and clarity. Based on many factors they either become gems or are used in industry for such items as saw blades and heavy drill bits.

Though not all diamonds become jewelry, they are diamonds nonetheless. The diamond that makes it to jewelry grade has undergone great refinement.

Seeing people for the diamonds they were created to be, inspires us to treat everyone with respect. Some radiate beauty inside and out. Others can be equally admired for their firmness, stability, and strength.

The diamond metaphor also reveals how an astonishing jewel may still be surrounded by volcanic debris. Recognizing that hurt, disappointment, and missed opportunities can obscure something extremely valuable; we may just need to look harder to find the hidden gem. Every human being can be considered a diamond in one stage or another.

Carrying a Club

Imagine holding a big club within the core of your being. Created to be strong, each healthcare professional is a protector of his family, patients, community, country, and world.

Sometimes though, events outside of our control may make us feel beaten down, especially when we cross paths with patients, families, and coworkers who have also experienced life challenges that leave them shattered. For a nurse or healer, carrying a big club image allows us to be an advocate for others. It provides strength enough to protect ourselves and others from individuals with low self-esteem or a poor attitude. As we cultivate a deep strength and resilience within our own being, it can be activated on behalf of others.

Of course, we don't want to walk around hitting others over the head or bashing them with words or deeds, but that big club image represents an internal strength used to intercede for what is right and good. Carrying a big club image allows each healthcare professional to be a champion for those who need one.

Shoveling in Spades

In gardening and industry, a spade is used to excavate earth and create a nurturing environment for growth. So, too, in healthcare.

Rarely does anyone trust others enough, nor are they comfortable enough to share their stories within the first few minutes of an encounter or even within the first few meetings. Often a healthcare professional is required to "dig deep" to discover truth and gain understanding. Listening closely and asking meaningful questions is essential to finding out what is at the heart of situations with our patients, their families, and our colleagues.

For most of us, truth is multilayered and deeply entrenched. It may even be crusted over with a rock-hard exterior to the point that an individual may not know her own truth or the cause of her pain and distress. As healthcare practitioners, bringing a spade to work helps us patiently excavate a deeper understanding of disease and lament of illness. The spade allows us to better provide cures and healing.

Have a Heart

Always, always, always—bring your heart to work! That alone sets healthcare professionals apart and makes us the special, unique individuals we are. It's most likely the reason we're in healthcare in the first place. Unfortunately, hearts can become calloused, scarred, and unfeeling, so it's up to us to be certain we keep them strong and healthy. And, sometimes that's not easy.

Setting hearts free to love depends on leaving them open to hurt. That means others may break them! Yet, the human heart has the incredible ability for every cardiac cell to beat independently. A heart contains untold numbers of cardiac cells. So even when it gets stepped on, ignored, or is broken—the heart has a limitless capacity to heal itself. Sometimes it takes a conscious decision to give our hearts the freedom to help us become the kind and loving healers we were destined to be.

In L. Frank Baum's *The Wonderful Wizard of Oz*, the Wizard tells the Tin Man: "Hearts will never be practical until they can be made unbreakable!" But Dorothy reassures the Tin Man, "A heart is not judged by how much you love, but how much you are loved by others." Finally, the Tin Man realizes he is willing to risk whatever is needed in order to truly have a heart. As the story nears its conclusion, the Tin Man understands the time has come for Dorothy to go back to Kansas. Dorothy leaves her friends in Oz, to which the Tin Man declares: "Now I know I have a heart; it is breaking!"

The final, most important lesson from a deck of cards, is simply do not hold your heart back from loving outrageously. Hearts—they're the best medicine you can give another person.

Recommended Resources

The Framework – Throughout History, It's All in the Cards

Hargrave, Catherine Perry. *A History of Playing Cards* (Mineola, NY: Dover, 2000).

Lesson 1 - Rules Change: Cards Don't

Centers for Medicare & Medicaid services (CMS).

Gallup. See https://news.gallup.com/poss.1654/Honesty-Ethics-Professions.aspx/

Institute of Medicine—a subsidiary of IHI.

Institute of Healthcare Improvement.

Joint Commission.

Norman, J., 2016. *Americans health care providers high on the honesty, ethics.* Washington, DC: Gallup. Retrieved from http//www.galllup.com/poll/200057/americans-rate-healthcare-providers-high-honesty-ethics.aspx/

Lesson 2 – You Can't Cure Everyone: You Can Heal Many

Alexander, Wil. *A Certain Kind of Light.* Video Documentary. Innerweave, (Loma Linda, CA: Loma Linda University Press, 2008)

Allenbaugh, Eric. Deliberate *Success* (Franklin Lakes, New Jersey: Career Press, Inc., 2002)

Berk, Lee S. *Mind, Body, Spirit: Exploring the Mind, Body, Spirit Connection through Research on Mirthful Laughter* (Hawthorne, NJ: Hawthorne Press, 2004).

Bridges, William. *Managing Transitions—Making the Most of Change* (Philadelphia: DeCapo Press: 2003, 2009).

Cousins, Norman. *Anatomy of an Illness* (New York: W. W. Norton & Co., 2005)

Kotter, John and Holger Rathgeber. *Our Iceberg is Melting* (New York: St. Martins Press, 2006)

Kubler-Ross, Elizabeth. *On Death and Dying* (New York: Random House, 1997).

Lesser, Elizabeth. *Broken Open* (Villard, NY: Simon and Schuster, 2008).

Meet Joe Black. Universal Pictures, 1998. Martin Brest, Director. Starring Brad Pitt and Anthony Hopkins

Wheatley, Margaret J. *Leadership and the New Science* (San Francisco: Berrett-Koehler, 2006).

Lesson 3—Every Card is Valuable: A Full Deck of Gifts

Damania, Zubin. www.zdoggmd.com

National Patient Safety Foundation—Institute for Healthcare Improvements.

National Patient Safety Goals.

Lesson 4 – Integrity: Determine to be a Great Player Instead of a Cheat

Agency for Healthcare Research and Quality.

Heinrich, Herbert William. *Industrial Accident Prevention: A Scientific Approach* (New York: McGraw-Hill, 1931)

Institute of Medicine.

Institute for Healthcare Improvement.

Institute for Safe Medication Practices.

National Quality Forum.

Lesson 5 – Claim Your ACE: Building A Bank of Skills

Brown, Brene. *Rising Strong* (New York: Spiegel & Grau, 2015)

Buckingham, Marcus. *Standout 2.0* (Boston: Harvard Business Press Review, 2015)

Lictenberg, Ronna. *Pitch Like a Girl* (Emmaus, PA: Rodale, 2005)

Ruiz. *The Four Agreements* (San Rafael, CA Amber-Allen, 2008)

Scumaci, Dondi. *Designed for Success* (Lake Mary, FL: Excels, 2004)

Lesson 6—A Poker Face Has Its Place

Chapman, Erie. *Radical Loving Care* (Nashville: Vaughan, 2009)

Frampton, Susan, and Patrick Charmel. *Putting Patients First—Best Practices in Patient Centered Ca*re (San Francisco: Jossey-Bass, 2009)

Lesson 7—Shuffle the Deck: Accepting Change and Discovering Opportunities

Collins, Jim. *Good to Great* (New York: Harper Collins, 2001).

Rath, Tom. *Strength Finders 2.0* (New York: Gallup, 2007).

Walsch, Neale Donald. *When Everything Changes* (Ashland, OR: EmNin, 2009)

Lesson 8—Close to the Vest or Face Up: Effective Communication

TeamSTEPPS. www.ahrq.gov.

Patterson, et al. *Crucial Conversations,* (New York: McGraw Hill, 2002)

Lesson 9 – Every Day Life Deals a New Hand: Developing Resilience

Shugart, Sandy. *Leadership in the Crucible of Work* (Maitland, FL: Florida Hospital Publishing, 2013)

Lesson 10—Remember the Suits: Treating People Well and Respecting Their Journey

Lee, Fred. *If Disney Ran Your Hospital* (Bozeman, MT: Second River Healthcare Press, 2004)

Tillquist, Kristin. *Capitalizing on Kindness* (Franklin Lakes, NJ: Career Press,

2009)

HAZEL CURTIS, RN, MPH

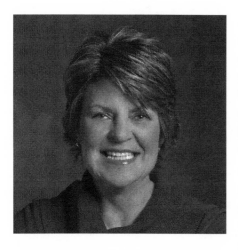

An "in demand" speaker, author, and leadership coach; Hazel has over four decades of experience in the healthcare industry. She spent her early nursing career in emergency and home healthcare. It has been Hazel's privilege to have worked the last two decades as a staff developer where she successfully launched leadership curriculum for frontline leaders to the C-Suite in a variety of healthcare organizations. Passionate about the employee and patient experience, Hazel supports leaders as they meet the challenges of creating a culture of safe, compassionate care.

After graduating with a BSN from Union College in Lincoln, NE, Hazel later received an MPH with emphasis in Health Education from Loma Linda University. Recently she completed a pre-doctoral leadership certification and holds lifetime credentials as an Allenbaugh Executive Coach.

Hazel's teaching and speaking career began in the mid-70s when she was asked to develop and instruct the paramedic program for the Loma Linda University School of Medicine. The paramedic program was in its infancy and yet to be offered in Inland Empire of Southern California. Standing in front of a room full of firemen gave powerful meaning to the words, "trial by fire!" That experience molded Hazel into a top-notch communicator.

As a leadership coach, keynote speaker, and training consultant; Hazel is passionate about transforming with intention, building people by building leaders. Even more, she wants to, inspire women to unleash passion, purpose, and power.

If you enjoyed this book and would like to find out more about Hazel Curtis, speaking dates, and other available resources, please visit www.hazelcurtis.com. At the website you'll be able to connect with Hazel through her blog, mastermind mentoring, and coaching resources. You will find a wealth of tools and information designed to help you succeed in providing care that nourishes your soul.

Along with being an accomplished author and coach, Hazel Curtis is also an exciting and motivating keynote speaker who travels the globe speaking to the needs of her audience. While sharing her dynamic and entertaining stories, Hazel helps her audience see themselves and their work more clearly. She offers wisdom and enthusiasm to professionals, hospitals and healthcare organizations. If you are interested in having Hazel speak to your organization, please go to www.hazelcurtis.com for details on booking information and available dates.

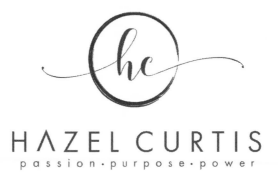

HAZEL CURTIS
passion · purpose · power

39092255R00087

Made in the USA
Middletown, DE
14 March 2019